MEMORY KEEPER FOR TWO

Journal of a Caregiver

By
Madeline J. McLean

Order this book online at www.trafford.com
or email orders@trafford.com

Most Trafford titles are also available at major online book retailers.

Print information available on the last page.

ISBN: 978-1-4120-3347-3 (sc)

Trafford rev. 05/18/2022

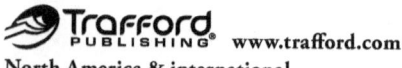 www.trafford.com

North America & international
toll-free: 844-688-6899 (USA & Canada)
fax: 812 355 4082

Table of Contents

Dedication

To my partner in life
who didn't deserve the ravages of this disease,
thank you for so many love-filled years.

Golden Years with Alzheimers

Window seat for eventide
Sad song of sunset
Dreams for the two of us
Forever unmet.

On the trail to twilight time
Shadows growing longer
Scatter the garden
The season is over.

Loved one seems far and away
Within reach but out of touch
Mate is memory keeper for two
And caregiver, and crutch.

MJMcLean

Acknowledgments

For insisting I tell my story, my thanks to Dr. Sharon Yoder who has been a creative partner in this project. And to all my children and grandchildren, thank you for your encouragement and ideas along the way. A special thanks to Jamie Yoder for producing my artwork for this book.

Part I

IN THE BEGINNING

"The grand essentials of happiness are something to do, something to love, and something to hope for."

Allan K. Chalmers

Chapter 1

ALL ABOUT US

Mac and I had each gone to college with another person in mind for a future marriage. My roommate had observed that I was missing some of the fun parties and with the aid of her frequent date, arranged a blind date for me with Mac-just so we would not miss a fun part of college life.

Our double date with my roommate and friend, turned out to be a "bug party". The fraternity members were to construct a bug for a race to the finish line. The rules stated no high tech mechanisms and this became a challenge for the engineers who were members of this fraternity and very much interested in "high tech".

Mac chose to carve some balsa wood into the shape of an ant and then painted it with many wild colors. There were a couple of axles and wheels, and in the tail of the insect he drilled a hole to hold a CO_2 charge—the kind that you buy at the drugstore in a sealed metal canister. When the charge was punctured, the ant flew down the track. It took a little time to puncture the hole while the other racers were rolling down the track, but once accomplished....we were at the finish line. Of course, Mac's "bug" won the race and for many years as we lived on both coasts of this country, I carried this little bug when we moved.

Then came the "Prohibition party" and my room-mates helped me dress for this one with someone providing black fishnet stockings and someone else providing the rose to wear behind one ear. Mac arrived at the dorm in his "gangster" suit with the baggy pants held in place by suspenders and with a gold chain pocket watch draped across his vest.

When we arrived at our destination, we were required to climb into the basement of the house via the basement window and slide down the coal chute. We danced to tunes of the twenties and thirties, and my drug of choice for the evening was caffeine in the colas I drank. We were drunk on fun. Are there any parties like this anymore?

We arrived back at the dorm just before curfew time and my roommate asked if I had a good time. We still laugh at my answer because I told her I had just met the man I was going to marry! Not sure why that popped out my mouth, but Mac and I continued to attend the fraternity parties as "friends" and discovered that when we were with each other, we were always in our comfort zone. I married my best friend.

Chapter 2

MORE ABOUT US

An English Heritage

As the oldest boy in a family of five boys, Mac had that special place of being the first grandchild on both sides of his family. His father had immigrated from the Isle of Mann and met Mac's mother who had descended from Pennsylvania Dutch immigrants.

His father was a finish carpenter and plied his trade with great skill. His mother, raised on a farm, became not only a first-rate cook but knew all the homemaking skills that are important to a comfortable family life. They interacted with the extended family at reunions, birthdays, and holidays. His parents belonged to various community clubs and service organizations. The boys were active in sports and had ponies and access to other pets as their father owned a pet store as a side business. Mac's family was a loving, conservative Midwestern family with all the traditional values of the time.

His parents left this life early, however. Mac's mother received the diagnosis of breast cancer in her early fifties. It progressed to her lungs and brain. His father had severe heart problems and he died a few years after Mac's mother had passed away. Most of Mac's aunts and uncles lived to see their seventies and were competent mentally at the time of their death. Combined with the fact that Mac's parents died early, we have no history of dementia of any kind recorded for the family.

Mac and his brothers became orphans when their own families were young. Since Mac was the oldest, we felt responsible for keeping the family unit intact when it came time for holidays such as Christmas and the Fourth of July. We usually held the picnic or dinner at our house and my sisters-in-law contributed by bringing dishes to the meal.

I think Mac felt it important that he play a "big brother" role whenever a younger brother of his had a problem where Mac thought he could help. We babysat occasionally for various brothers, and provided finances if there was a need and we were in a position to do so. Mac is very proud of his brothers and their accomplishments and had liked to recount early stories when all five boys lived at home.

With a father from English heritage, however, conversations and communications were never on a very intimate level. Feelings and emotions were kept in check. The loudest I ever heard any of the brothers speak was if their team scored while watching a baseball game.

The brothers enjoyed sports of all kinds, being spectators and participating. I cannot remember ever hearing Mac or his brothers swear and anger shown only on their countenance, rarely in their behaviors. This pattern continued while each was raising his children. In thirty plus years of marriage, I could probably not count to ten times

I knew Mac to be irate. Alzheimer's has changed the pattern.

All About Me

Just as Mac grew up in a typical middleclass Midwestern community, I too had grown up in a very small rural town.

The population of our little town was close knit and caring about their community and looked out for all the children.

My father was the local superintendent of the public school and my mother was an elementary teacher in the same system. My only sibling was four years younger than I was and I enjoyed being the oldest child in our family unit as well as being the oldest grandchild on my father's side.

After graduation from high school, I attended one of the big ten schools hoping to graduate after the usual four years and embark on the career of my choice. It was while attending the university that I met Mac on the blind date.

My growing up was in the best of times –the fifties— reminiscent of drive-ins, saddle shoes, and Elvis. Times were good economically after the deprivation of the war years, and I grew up with the belief that being loyal to the American flag, being strong in the faith of my choice, listening to Mom and Dad, and appreciating apple pie and baseball would ensure me of a good chance at happiness.

I brought to the marriage expectations like many women of the fifties. I hoped to marry the man of my choice, raise a family, and prepare for a career if I chose to work outside the home. It became harder work than I had envisioned, but it met most of my expectations. I believed the "golden years" after retirement would be the best years yet. Nothing could have prepared me for the challenges I have had to face in confronting Alzheimer's disease as it has victimized my spouse.

During forty years of marriage and five children, life was normal, up times and down times, as all couples have.

Mac and I had divided work in the marriage and in the home and business. Mac worked for himself having an engineering practice that employed from three to twelve people at one time. He worked long hours and kept track of our retirement accounts, our insurances and long-term goals while I managed the daily household accounts and children's schedules. I also had a small counseling practice. Things were going smoothly.

After I retired from my counseling practice, Mac was trying to wrap things up with his business so he could retire also. We were enjoying the five children and the spouses of those that were married and best of all, eight grandchildren. We attended recitals, the ball games, and band concerts as often as we could and enjoyed them all. Mac and I traveled some, but we were busy thinking about retirement and what changes it would make in our lives.

One day after babysitting with Corey, one of my grandsons, I came home with such a shoulder ache. It continued to ache and radiated into my ear. The next day I was not much better and on the way to have a dresser refinished, I just stopped the car and told Mac he would have to drive me to the doctor...the pain was getting much worse.

After our family doctor ran an EKG, he called an ambulance as he felt I was having a mild heart attack. Angioplasty and three stents later, I came home with instructions for a new lifestyle. After a heart attack, most people suffer depression and a lot of fear. Mac was there for me staying up with me when I could not sleep and driving me around when I became restless. The family was focusing on my health problems and me, and at the time, Mac seemed to be functioning fine.

Retirement, we agreed, would be pretty much continuing enjoying the family as we had been doing with perhaps a little more travel thrown in. We had thought that perhaps we would continue to develop some of our hobbies, like making woodcrafts and perhaps even becoming a vendor at some craft fairs. Mac liked doing woodworking and I enjoyed painting and needlecrafts.

We had even thought we would enjoy our travel trailer and had it outfitted just the way we wanted to accommodate us best for long and short stays...maybe even the winter in the South, especially since my daughter and her husband lived there. There were relatives in the West and Northwest that we planned on visiting.

Mac had thought he would like to take some woodworking classes in furniture making and I had thought Comparative Religion and Anthropology classes at a university might be fun. Perhaps I could even sign up for an archeology dig. We were both serious about doing some volunteer work for Habitat for Humanity. There was no shortage of ideas or possibilities for our retirement days. So I had experienced a little setback in the health realm. I was doing fine and with a few modifications in my lifestyle, things would continue as planned.

Chapter 3

OUR CHILDREN

Life Is A Bowl of Jelly

Brian is our oldest son, who thought you could wiggle and giggle through life and not take things too seriously. I had always thought he would marry the little floozy who sat on the fender of the car, smoking her cigarette and wearing her miniskirt. Brian's siblings kept telling me I was so wrong—Brian would marry an audience.

And then, along came Deb—a daughter-in-law every mother wishes for. She was practical ("I always read the directions and follow them"), feet on the ground, methodical and goal oriented besides being the loving mother of three and of course, Brian's audience of one.

They lived in the state capital where Deb became a vice president of one of our nation's largest banks while Brian worked in retail management. They lived busy lives involved in their work, and their children,--two girls in high school and a son in his first year of college.

The children dutifully called once a week and drove the three hours for a visit whenever they could. Then I informed them of the "diagnosis".

At first, Brian told me that "everyone forgets now and then" and Dad has had a lot of stress with me being sick and all. Of the abnormal behaviors, Brian could rational-ize every one of them. This was first-rate denial but with time, he is learning to cope.

The grandchildren have been more accepting of the facts. The youngest daughter did a research assignment on Alzheimer's disease and called me for some input. She received an A+ on her report and her class asked ques-tions for twenty minutes. Her teacher told her it was the most impressive report she had ever had submitted in her classes.

The older brother, in his first year of college, recog-nized a gold mine when he saw one and decided to use the same subject for a research paper of his own. Being very nice to his little sister, he used her paper for reference. Having a relative living with this disease personalized both papers for the grandchildren.

Brian's oldest daughter has just given us our first great grandchild…a little, little girl with a head full of curls. I told Mac that Haley had arrived and she would be our first great grandchild. He had just a blank stare, and of course, did not know who these people were. Another joy I cannot share and a little girl whose antics will not be appreciated by a great grandfather who has enjoyed all his grandchildren in the past.

Alzheimer's does not fit into the "Life is a Bowl of Jelly" philosophy as Brian and family are slowly learning. Brian knows this is eventually a terminal disease.

Life Is A Gourmet Buffet

When our second son arrived, we knew from the be-ginning his philosophy on life—snap to, on the double!

He loved a schedule. His meals were to be on time, a bath before bed, and diapers were to be dry. Life is a gourmet buffet and Bret would sample what life had to offer with a little taste of many things, but banquet fare please,--no hasty puddings.

He decided upon engineering as a major in college and a company who had projects in the South hired him after graduation. After savoring the South and his job there was finished, Bret decided an MBA was in order. He graduated cum laude and opted to forage Europe for some international fare. He worked four years in Germany at an Air Force base. Eventually the base became one of those scheduled for closing, and letters and phone calls from home alerted Bret that something was wrong with Dad. He decided to come back to USA and see if he could help in the family business.

The miles away from the scene at home had given him perspective that other family members could not imagine.

Bret felt the time had come to close down the business. After the diagnosis, siblings thought Bret harsh in wanting to finalize the business, get finances in order, and face reality.

Bret has probably been the least in denial of all the children. All the time he has told me not to count on him for any caretaking… "I am not a caretaker, I just don't do that" has been his mantra.

However, this is the person who calls each day. This person went with me to the lawyer's office and to court when the need arose. This person read contracts, hired roofers, and negotiated the lowest possible price for my car. Bret, with an aptness beyond my qualifications, dealt with the stockbrokers...things I had never expected I would have to do.

Rosemary has recently appeared in Bret's life softening the edges a bit. All the family loves her and she has at one point in her life, taken care of an Alzheimer's victim. She knows our dilemma of losing a loved one to a brain-wasting disease. She will ease Bret into the realization that what he contributes to relieve the stress of daily confrontations makes him a "caretaker" after all, and one of the best.

A Meat and Potatoes Kind of Guy

Our middle child was a gift to Mac and me-- unplanned, with an easy pregnancy and birth. He was an easygoing baby and little boy, always "going with the flow". He grew up to be very tall in a house of short people. Our family teddy bear was a meat and potatoes kind of guy, not too impressed with flash, and very accepting of life however it was presented on his platter.

He was a first-rate student and shined in the sports of his choice. Brad had few wants in life—a musket loading gun, a good tennis racquet, a pick-me-up truck, and Lori.

Brad decided to join the Air Force, became a specialist in an obscure foreign language, and married his perfect love match before going overseas. Brad and Lori had two girls that have survived monumental physical problems and have thrived. Kadie entered this world the size of her father's hand weighing in at two pounds. Last year she participated in the United States Olympics as a torchbearer. Brad and Lori are the perfect parents and their daughters have grown into loving, caring and achieving young women.

Then, along came Michael, a perfectly mischievous little boy who thinks he has three mothers with the older girls in the house, and believes he should be hunting and fishing, riding a motorcycle popping wheelies and driving a car like his Dad. Michael is four, going on twenty.

Brad has always worked in the field of construction—either in project management or in engineering, sometimes in the family business. Brad looked askance at his father's strange behaviors when they occurred, and until the diagnosis, I think he dealt with them on a one by one basis. Perhaps he did not want to believe they were a symptom of something greater than stress, normal forgetfulness, or miscommunication.

After the doctors diagnosed Mac, Brad, back from the military service, was there to help on a personal basis. He was grateful to know that there was a reason for the progression of his Dad's problems. Brad is very busy with his own growing family, and the fact that he works out of town, makes time limited for him to deal with our problems.

From the very first, Brad has offered to build us a suite or small house to accommodate our needs and likings. He has suggested he build this next door to his family so he and his wife can be there to help us. Brad understands my needs for independence and yet the needs for security in taking care of his father. Brad repeats his offer and we know it is genuine. Therefore, while on a day-to-day basis Brad cannot check in, the family teddy bear offers security in the long-term area of insecurity that is part of this disease.

Hi, Red

We moved to the new house at Christmastime and I promptly came down with the flu....but the flu stayed around for nine months, and then, Rory was born. And what a fun kid! Short in stature, but big in ideas and opinions, and not afraid to voice them from the minute he could utter words. Rory was always busy, way too busy to pick up his clothes, or put away his toys. He was forming this group or that and eventually formed this company or that. School was for the most part a place for "networking". Rory has been a disc jockey, a commercial photographer, a landscaper, a roofer, and has worked in the family business. Rory turned the blueberries growing in our back yard into a worthy cordial. Never was there an idle moment in this man's kitchen.

Then he found the little girl with the very long name and the very big brown eyes. They celebrated birthdays on the same day in summer, and soon they wed. Their little girl was born two years later and she was tiny, dainty, and so prim. She, too, found that her voice could be effective early on and now spends a lot of time teaching her parents the proper way of parenting and pointing out the error of their ways. She is seven.

Two years later a little boy was born who had his mother's big doe-like eyes and the longest lashes to shade them. He received a diagnosis of mild autism about the age of two and the family compares the symptoms of autism to that of Alzheimer's disease. The gene studies on my grandson were done but gene research has not been completed on Alzheimer's disease. The retreat into worlds unknown to us...the blank stares...the trouble speaking thoughts... we wonder if there is a link.

Rory works as a project manager with a large company that needs him to live closer to his work. Soon he won't be a stone's throw away to help me hunt Mac if he decides to wander and evade me. Rory is active in organizations for autism and works at the state level. He tells me we will try for caregivers' grants of which this state and country has few. Rory knows firsthand the stresses put upon caregivers with seventy percent of them ending with health problems of their own.

Rory, who has never had a nickname, came into our house the other morning and Mac said, "Hi, Red". We will miss Rory and his family when they move.

I Found The Twinkies

Raising the boys was fun but Mac and I had always wondered what it would be like to have a little girl. Nine months after applying to adopt a little girl, the phone rang and the social worker asked us to bring clothes for a baby to wear coming home from the hospital. I couldn't remember what all that entailed, so I called my Mom who rushed out to the store, bought the necessities, and hurried home to wash and dry them.

Mac and I brought home a three-day old infant that looked for all the world like a beautiful doll. She quickly captured her daddy's heart and became the darling of our family.

Early on, we knew Laurie would be the caretaker

type. She would try mothering her older brothers and left notes for Rory – "Clean up your Room", signed "Mother" – and would tack this on his bedroom door. Or, in the freezer she would put a note reading, "Ha, I found your Twinkies!"

The boys all enjoyed having this little fireball for a sister and the protective feelings have remained. I enjoyed having another female in our household to share shopping, share gabfests, and share making wedding plans.

Laurie married a chef whose home country is Germany and she has always resided many miles away. Nevertheless, that hasn't kept her from keeping in touch and involved in all the family decisions. Laurie knows when all you need is a listener, or when you would like a little sympathy, or if we need to take action.

As time went by, and her Dad's disease became more advanced, I found we had property that needed transferred and contracts that needed to be re-negotiated…things that Mac would have taken care of when he was well. I was not sure how to progress and these things seemed bogged down in minutiae. Laurie would make the phone calls that got things moving and resolved. Problem-solving and motivating people to take action are talents of hers.

Thank goodness for E-mail and telephones. Laurie checks in every day by electronic mail and calls home at least once or twice per week. She also checks with her brothers that live close by us in order to get a better perspective on the situation in our house.

She has a husband that supports her in her efforts to do what she can with the distance that is between us.

Denial has never been descriptive of Laurie—action and involvement best describe this daughter of ours. She is one of the main pillars of my support system and I could not do without this little mover and shaker.

Chapter 4

A BOISTEROUS BUNCH

Christmas Past, Christmas Present

Christmas in our house was a big noisy holiday. All year I bought little gifts for the five children and stored them at my mother's house. When Christmas arrived, I wrapped all gifts, even the sidewalk chalk and coloring books. The room was full of the Christmas tree and gifts. On the mantel were the stockings including the ones for the dog and cat. These are the memories Mac has lost and I cannot share with him.

As the children became adults with children of their own, we also added little games or acts of entertainment you were required to perform before you could open your gifts.

One year, Brad and family taught us all how to do a turkey call when hunting for wild turkeys. (How often would we be doing that?) The same year, Rory and family put on little Santa hats they had made and sang carols (his children were toddlers and it was their first performance of Jingle Bells). Everyone had an act. Memories, again lost for Mac.

In our family, allergies were a big problem. There were special diets and at one point, could not include eggs for one child, citrus for another, and milk products for another. About this time, we discovered pies as a dessert that everyone could enjoy. So pies have been included as part of all our holiday treats for this family.

One Christmas, Mac and I made a video for each family. Flour on our faces and all, we showed how to make an apple pie. I am not sure Mac would recognize anyone on the tape.

Last year our daughter and husband were home from Florida for the holidays. Laurie made sure there was a gift from Dad for me under the tree. Mac, of course, did not realize he was giving me a gift.

The children never used to ask what they could buy Dad for Christmas. They chose things for his hobbies, or perhaps for the sports he enjoyed. Now they are puzzled. Dad cannot read, nor participate in hobbies or sports, and his days are spent moving things from one position to another or pacing the floor. I do not know what to tell them.

My birthday, Mother's Day, Father's Day, and our anniversary will pass and I will not mention them because Mac does not know what the celebrations are. On some days, he may tell you he is not married and has no children. Most days he knows my name, but there are days when he is not sure. Most of the time he thinks I am his sister.

The family will continue to celebrate the "big" holidays and, perhaps on some level, Mac will appreciate the family being together, or remember the celebration.

The "Back Forty"

Mac and I both had grandmothers who lived on farms. My grandmother took me with her grocery shopping one time I remember so vividly. Grandma was shocked when all she had purchased was some flour, sugar, and cheese and it came to almost three dollars!

Grandma had a garden, an orchard, cows, pigs, chickens, and woods that grew wild grapes and nut trees. She knew what to do with these "raw materials" and had a cellar with a dirt floor that housed a running spring in a cement trough. She kept her root vegetables and apples for winter storage in the cellar, along with the cream and butter in the spring-fed trough. My grandfather had an icehouse where he placed cut ice from the creek during the winter storing it in sawdust.

Along about the Fourth of July, Grandma invited the family to make homemade ice cream to use the leftover ice. These were the big five-gallon ice cream makers with a crank, and the men sat in the shade of the elm trees where they talked and cranked the cream into ice cream that would make Ben and Jerry proud.

These memories for me have added to the obsession of making food from the "raw materials", at least part of the time. I wanted our children to know how you make strawberry jam, sauerkraut, and yogurt cheese.

Every year our family would make it a point to pick our strawberries from the truck farm's nearby strawberry fields. One year we let the boys climb the trees at a commercial farm to pick cherries. It had rained the night before. The leaves were wet, and so were the boys' clothes by the time they had finished. While seeding each one of those ruby red little gems, we voted that next year, we would buy our cherries already picked!

Our "back forty" contained forty or so blueberry bushes. Mac would help with the netting and picking of two hundred or more quarts the patch yielded when it was in its prime. He seemed to enjoy being a "farmer in the city" and there were always nets to mend and bushes to trim.

Ironically, blueberries are the one food research is studying as a food that perhaps might have enough antioxidants to prevent or delay Alzheimer's disease. Blueberries have not prevented the disease from taking Mac victim.

Are We There Yet?

In Mac's family, they spent vacation time working around their home, and possibly taking the vacation days during the date of the family reunion. My parents were schoolteachers and summer vacations usually meant an auto trip sightseeing in one of our then, forty-eight states.

When Mac and I married, there were very different ideas about vacation time. I eventually convinced him that vacations away from home could be fun, and conceded that vacations could be fun spent in one spot such as a resort.

The two of us were able to experience family vacations as well as time away for just the two of us. Some of our favorite recesses from daily work were visiting out of this country and enjoying other cultures. At one time when the children were small, we enjoyed camping in a little tent camper we owned. We dreamed then about purchasing the perfect trailer for traveling when we retired.

Eventually we ordered that perfect trailer made to the specifications we thought would be perfect for traveling and perhaps spending a few months away from Midwest winters.

Shortly after the delivery of our dream trailer, Mac became hesitant about pulling it although we had a heavy vehicle to do so.

In the first two or three years we owned the trailer, Mac and I used it to vacation only two weeks. The rest of the time, it sat in storage, or parked as an additional bedroom at our home when we had large numbers of visiting guests.

I was puzzled the whole time as to why, when Mac had poured over the various floor plans for trailers right beside me, and he had worked in the building and engineering fields his whole life, he could not figure out how to hook up the trailer to campsite facilities.

I was so disappointed that he found this idea of traveling a nightmare in reality. How could I have read his reactions so erringly about these plans we had worked on for so long?

Mac gave me no answers. In fact, he just did not answer my questions.

The beginning of Alzheimer's had probably already begun to rear its ugly head in the form of confusion, and fear of anything new or unfamiliar. I was very much unprepared to lose one of the precious memory makers of our life together—our vacation experiences.

We had fun tales to tell from every vacation or trek that we took, such as the vacation to one of the Caribbean islands. A seatmate on the plane asked where we were going. She lived on the island and when I told her the name of the resort, she loudly told everyone within hearing distance that in the islands it was called "That Menopausal Manor". Still in my forties, I decidedly did not appreciate that!

Mac shows no recollection of any of the vacation times, and one wonders how memorable must an event be to remain in your memory forever. The word – vacation- has now taken on a new meaning for me. It now refers to a day or two away from constant care giving.

Respite care is very expensive even if it is available in the area in which you live. When you add the cost of taking your patient to a facility, which must have a specialized secured wing for Alzheimer's patients for insurance purposes, the vacation days can become financially prohibitive.

While you can find daycare workers to come into your home, again, twenty-four hours care is affordable for only a few. Most workers will be prepared to take only eight-hours shifts. This is confusing for the Alzheimer's victim who thrives better in a known routine with familiar faces. Family members who are probably giving already as much time and effort as they can, will find vacationing for the primary caregiver extremely burdensome.

Our last vacation was to a time-share on a lovely coast in the South. It is a place we had taken a week or two for nearly twenty years. Last fall a friend accompanied us to help me with Mac and enjoy the scenery with us. It sounded like a good plan and nothing happened that was unusual.

Nevertheless, in your mind is always the specter of the ghost of Alzheimer's and the question, will it affect Mac's behaviors. You are also constantly making adjustments to accommodate the disease. A truly relaxing vacation is out of reach.

New horizons to explore and distant lands to discover are now just a dream for one partner of this marriage and a blank screen for the other.

May I Have This Dance?

When our children became more independent, I felt that Mac and I should start sharing more things as a couple. Perhaps we could find a hobby or sport that we could both enjoy. My idea of the perfect sport was a rocking chair on an old porch, curled up with a good "whodunit", and a glass of iced tea, which certainly did not fit Mac's idea of the perfect sport!

We finally decided that I would try golfing with him. I had taken a golf course as part of my physical education requirement in college and I had been taught stances, swings, and observing others. We never played a game!

However, I aced the course and thought, "How hard can this be".

Mac cooperated by bringing home a set of women's clubs and mentioning that he had reserved a tee time for us on Wednesday morning. We started out bright and early. Two and a half hours later, we were one-third through the course. By this time, Mac was encountering doctors, dentists, and other acquaintances that played on Wednes-days, and becoming more uneasy by the minute.

When we arrived home that day, Mac gave the clubs to our son, Bret, telling him he didn't think I would be needing them anymore! Fine with me as the mystery shelves at the library looked more and more enticing.

After the children were in high school and in college, Mac and I next decided to enroll in some dance lessons. We waltzed, jitterbugged, and square danced into some competitions. We met so many fun new friends and won some of those competitions complete with trophies and pictures.

This was also a fun way to stay fit. This became our "couple time".

The staff at the daycare center tells me that Mac loves to dance. When the center invited spouses and friends for a Father's Day/Mother's Day luncheon, there was a deejay. The clients, who were able, were dancing. The Sisters told me that Mac had been dancing an hour before I arrived. He mostly moved swaying to the music and if he had a partner, twirled her round and round.

Staff has suggested when Mac becomes agitated at home try playing the dance music. I have done so but Mac doesn't seem to respond.

He had always watched the Lawrence Welk program on Saturday nights and would sit, watching and keeping time to the music. At this stage of the disease, he seems disinterested and walks away from the room where the program is playing. "Couple time" is just a memory for me alone.

Part II

THE DIAGNOSIS

When Albert Einstein was serving as proctor for a university test, a student raised his hand and said, "Sir, I think there's been a mistake. This is the same test we were given last year." Einstein replied, "Yes, the test is the same as last year, but this year the answers are different."

Chapter 5

PUZZLES APPEAR

Ten or twelve years ago, unusual things began to happen in the family business, and in our family life. One of the first things we noticed about Mac was some business decisions that lost us money. He would sign his name on commitments that were iffy at best.

He always had the excuse that he had relied on some misinformation. I remember at the time being puzzled, and I am ashamed to admit, wondering about Mac's intelligence level and his denial that he was the cause of any problems.

We had always taken the children to Florida in the spring during their vacation. We would rent a cottage on the beach near a town where our relatives lived. Since we had gone to this area for twelve to fifteen years, it was a familiar area to drive. The last time we went for a visit, I was surprised that Mac was very lost, and did not remember the highways.

He had a hard time locating our relatives' home and one time made a left turn from the wrong lane. For an engineer who always knew directions, always knew where he was, and a driver of the most careful sort, these unusual behaviors sent up some red flags.

A year or two later, when we went to visit our daughter and her husband, Mac arose in the middle of the night, went to the bathroom, and started to shave. I questioned him as to what he was doing, and he appeared puzzled and confused. We were not due to leave for home for another day or two.

After a time, I noticed that he was using his lips when reading the newspaper in the evenings. A few months later, he began following along with his finger the lines he was reading. I queried him about his eyesight and he assured me it was fine. He did not seem to realize that this was a change in his behaviors nor strange in any way.

I asked my relatives if they had noticed anything different in Mac's behaviors and especially, his memory. One brother told me what he noticed was my constant answering for Mac or prompting him before Mac could answer on his own. I then began to question if perhaps I was the problem, and perhaps I was overreacting to events.

If, for instance, I wanted to inform Mac that I would not be home for lunch the next day because of a hairdresser appointment, I would have to start telling him three days beforehand. It seemed that if I could get the information into Mac's long-term memory bank, he would recall it. However, he had such a loss of short-term memory. For a time, in the office and at home, I relied on notes taped in strategic places.

Life kept going in this manner quite a few months. One summer morning I told Mac I would like to attend a dog show on the other side of town. He was not interested in going, so I left to attend on my own. I returned to the house two hours later and found Mac in great pain, and lying on the couch. He was very willing to go to the emergency room.

Doctors diagnosed Mac with pancreatic inflammation and admitted him to the hospital. He stayed there nearly a week. After doing exploratory tests using anesthesia, the family members who came to visit Mac noticed an immediate improvement in his memory problems. Mac was his old self.

After Mac came home and the effects of the anesthesia had disappeared from his body, all his memory problems returned. This, I have since learned, has been observed in other Alzheimer's patients.

Our family doctor informed of the situation, decided on a round of CAT scans, brain-wave tests, and any other laboratory tests that might give insight into the memory problem. Alzheimer's is essentially a diagnosis that occurs by the process of elimination. At the time, there was no test for positive diagnosis. The damage that occurs during this disease is visible only as the result of an autopsy after the patient has died. All of Mac's lab tests were negative.

The next step was a consultation at the Cleveland Clinic with a doctor who specialized in the diagnosis of dementia and, especially Alzheimer's disease. Mac drove to the hospital and experienced no problems in wandering among the maze of tall buildings that comprise Cleveland Clinic.

We were ushered into a small office with no equipment but furnished with a small desk and a few chairs. When the doctor entered the room, he first told us some facts about dementia. He related there were many kinds.

Some kinds are treatable and doctors are of help, and many kinds of dementia are diagnosed with laboratory tests. There are some that he could only diagnose by ruling out other types of dementia—diagnosis by exclusion.

The doctor began by asking Mac if he had been experiencing any problems with memory. Mac did not admit to this and began with his "excuses" for any problems he had been having. As I listened, I realized Mac was ailing much more than our family had realized.

The doctor asked about a new event—a devastating plane crash that had occurred and taken the life of one of our nation's prominent and promising young people. Mac and I had watched eight hours of news coverage the day before our appointment at the Cleveland Clinic. Mac's answer was he remembered a tragic plane crash that had occurred years before when an Olympic team was lost.

This mathematical whiz, this engineer who could work complex mathematical formulas without paper, when asked if he could count backwards from one hundred by seven's, could not. I was shocked with his not being able to follow instructions, and then, not being able to perform this task.

After asking Mac what day it was (it was Friday and Mac answered Tuesday), and asking Mac if he remembered what floor this office was on (Mac did not remember), the doctor left the room. I suppose these last questions were to test short-term memory.

When the doctor returned, he told us that he had ruled out the many other forms of dementia, and felt sure Mac had Alzheimer's disease. He said he was sorry to tell us there were few medications on the market that would help. He would give a report to our family doctor and perhaps he would prescribe Aricept, the only drug of prominence at this time. The doctor's last words were, "There is no need to return to Cleveland Clinic."

Neither of us was too shocked because we did not know much about Alzheimer's disease. I can remember thinking, "Oh, great! I hope Mac can find his way home because I surely don't know where I am."

Fit But Failing

In the early stages of Mac's disease, I noticed it was becoming harder and harder for him to make decisions. We were used to taking two or three meals per week in a restaurant.

First, I noticed Mac felt more comfortable in the restaurants that we frequented often. Our little town was known for the huge number of eating-places. There is always a new one to try but Mac seemed calmest in the places that we had eaten many times before.

Then he would say things like, "just order that for me too," or tell the waitress, "make that a double order." Later, he said nothing but just waited for me to order for the both of us. Sometimes he didn't know how to eat a particular food and would eat his sandwich with his fork. Over time it became obvious, he didn't want to touch his food with his fingers.

Occasionally I would have to stop him from wanting to gather up the dishes and take them with him when he left the restaurant table. He wanted to leave when he was finished eating and it was hard to keep him in his seat until our tab had been presented.

Now it is easier to just order and pick up so he can eat at home unless I have family that can go with us. Eating at home has it problems too sometimes. Mac went through a period when he said I was trying to poison him. And he would refuse to eat things that he had liked all his life.

In the beginning, there was an unexplained weight loss that the doctors spent a lot of time doing tests to see why it was happening. All tests were negative. I tried to present him with a varied diet and frequent snacks along with his meals. Eventually, the weight has been regained. Some patients start eating everything in sight and try to eat things that aren't edible. We have not experienced that problem.

Mac had always been good about drinking many fluids. That has become a problem for us as he either doesn't see the glass at mealtime and has to be reminded that his juice, water, or tea is there to drink, or he doesn't recognize thirst. He is now unable to get a drink from the faucet (he wouldn't know where the glasses were, or how to turn on the faucet) so I must remember to offer drinks.

Mac is unable to tell me what he had for lunch on the days he is at daycare so we perhaps have the same thing for dinner. Daycare gives him a snack (usually cookies and juice) in the morning and in the afternoon. They have a hot lunch for the clients, which is always soft food such as soup, sandwich, or chicken stew, applesauce or other cooked fruit.

In the support meeting, we learned that one man whose wife has Alzheimer's tells him every day that the daycare fed her that darned split pea soup again.

With Mac, my son and I noticed that he was craving sweets and if he ate too many, it seemed to make his memory symptoms worse. I asked our family doctor if there was a connection between sugar metabolism and Alzheimer's. He did not know of any but was willing to do a blood sugar test and that, again, turned out to be within the normal range. I have found that there is some new research being done on the sugar metabolism for these people and it has to do with a portion of the insulin response, with a gene being responsible for the problem. The leader of our support group had given us the information that since sweet is the strongest of all our taste senses, some researchers feel that sweet, the deepest groove of all taste sensations in our brain tissue, would be the last to go from our memory. It is obvious there is much more work to do in the research area.

Alzheimer's victims thrive on a routine, and even having company for a day stimulates them to the point where their behaviors can become trying.

I have learned that in addition to tangles and plaque in the brain of an Alzheimer's patient, there can be some growths called Lewy bodies, named after the Dr. Lewy who discovered them. And while the growths cannot be detected except with an autopsy, they have made a correlation between the patients that have Lewy bodies in the brain and those that exhibit psychotic behavior. Never have the children and I had to be afraid or cautious around Mac. But I have been warned by his doctors several times that he might in the blink of an eye exhibit violence and it could be towards me. I have been warned to call the paramedics for transport if Mac becomes ill or has a fever as that can bring on violence.

In the early stages I remember the first time I saw any of this behavior. The phone rang and for some unknown reason Mac grabbed it and threw it—my direction. I was so puzzled because it was so unlike him and I kept searching for the reason I had instigated that behavior.

Now I know, that it could be someone or something that only materializes for people that have Alzheimer's disease and isn't in our realm of reality.

This was one of the hardest lessons as a caregiver I had to learn for I hung onto the hope that the relationship between Mac and me was still a close, personal and intimate one. Alzheimer's changes that description.

Chapter 6

STRANGE HAPPENINGS

Mac had always been active in sports. He had ponies of his own, which he raced at the county fairs and because he was small of stature, he raced for other owners as well. He was an avid baseball player in high school and he ran track. In college, he started playing golf and continued this sport by joining golf leagues after we were married.

There were times in summer when I felt abandoned to babysitting for our children and resented the baseball games and golf outings which took Mac away from our family.

He enjoyed it so much he could not imagine why it was not a passion of mine.

Winter was the time for tennis. Mac enjoyed tennis under the "bubble" with his friendly foursome—the judge, the doctor, and the city official,--friends of his in this small town. Mac possessed a Napoleonic competitiveness that sometimes is present in persons of short stature. It was hard for him to play sports "just for fun." He passed the passion for these three sports to his sons who continue to play them throughout their busy lives. Some of his favorite times with the boys were the family golf outings. The first words when they returned were, "Well, Dad won again!"

The last time Mac played golf with his sons and brothers, he was unable to observe golf etiquette. He would pick up other persons' balls and play them, or he was unable to take turns at the tee. He lost his wallet and was sure someone at the course had taken it.

After brothers and sons hunted the golf cart and premises, and asked if anyone had found the wallet, one son came home and checked the bedroom. There he found the wallet, --on the dresser.

I think this was the first time Mac's brothers became cognizant of how bad the situation was and how Alzheimer's disease can disrupt even the best of times.

Playing the game was not fun anymore and became a series of irritations and confusion for the people playing with him. Along with his catcher's mitt, and his tennis racquet, Mac's golf clubs are stored in the garage.

The Portrait Is Missing

Our home has different levels and one day, when I was on the upper level, the telephone rang. I answered on a phone that is not portable so I was rather stuck in one spot.

I was chatting, looking round the room, and then I saw the bare square on the wall. This space housed our family portrait in an antique frame from my grandmother's attic.

It was so puzzling to me that Mac had gotten that big picture down and taken it away somewhere without me seeing him do it. After the phone call, I started searching.

Perhaps he had put it into a hall closet, or just carried it to another room. Asking an Alzheimer's patient about anything is an exercise in futility.

The longer I searched for the portrait, the more upset I became. Two weeks later, one of my sons needed something from the storage room over the garage. When he came into the house, Brad said I owed him major applause. Here Brad came with the portrait! Mac had hidden the family picture in a box behind some other furniture stored in the garage loft. I had not seen him leave the house with this picture even though the frame measures nearly two and a half feet square. We will never know why he took it down, or why he hid it.

Hiding things has been a big problem for the family. We have things missing that I have never found. I dare not leave my eyeglasses lying around. I own a couple of pairs and both must remain out of sight. My first pair disappeared and I have never recovered them.

One day I missed my spectacles and here Mac came walking in from the back yard wearing my glasses on top of his. This has happened more than once and Lens Crafters has had to realign and refit mine often.

Mac's wallet disappeared again after the golf outing and we have never found it. However, I had removed all credit cards but had let him carry the wallet because he prided himself in having his engineering license and drivers' license even though he was practicing neither. I thought we could perhaps use them for identification if Mac became lost.

Mac has had a fixation on his belts. Every night when he removes his clothes to retire, I hide his belt. Otherwise, he arises in the night and he may hide the belt where I cannot find it. I have found his belt in his golf ball storage bucket. I have found it in various dresser drawers in his bedroom. One time, I found it rolled and stuffed into an old shoe. So, I purchase belts in twos. The day after I had purchased two more, the brown one disappeared. I have never found it.

One morning while getting Mac dressed to go to the daycare center, I found his shoes were missing. After hunting for half an hour, I found one shoe on a dining room chair pushed under the table and out of sight, and the other shoe was in one of his dresser drawers. Now these shoes were in his closet when I put him into bed the previous evening.

Moreover, there are things that I really don't think he is hiding, but I don't understand just what is happening in his thinking process. I was doing some cleaning and handed Mac the broom and dustpan asking him if he would sweep our kitchen floor. I was thinking that this might keep him occupied while I finished other tasks. Not able, or either not wanting to do this little job, Mac put the broom across the doorway of the furnace room but the dustpan was missing. It wasn't in the cleaning closet, wasn't in the wastebasket, and I was unable to locate it the rest of that day. Next morning, I opened the kitchen knife drawer, and there was the dustpan, dirt and all, in the drawer.

As soon as Mac is finished eating, I must remove the dishes to the sink. If I didn't do this, he would pick up his dishes and we might find them anyplace. I have found them in the laundry room (was he mixed up as to what sink to put them in?), in the cabinet in the bathroom, (another sink error?), and in the bottom of the garbage bag—can't imagine about that one. Another time I couldn't find the silverware or his plate. I finally found the plate but hunted for the silverware for two days.

It was a snowy, icy day and on my entryway, I kept a salt sack to sprinkle on the sidewalk ice. Inside the sack was the silverware from Mac's meal two days previous.

Another day was a hot summer one and I had all the doors open. I thought Mac was still in the house, so I am not sure how much time had elapsed before I realized he had gone outside.

I looked up and down the street but didn't see him. I called his name inside the house and out. There was no answer. After going into the garage and happening to look up the stairs, I saw the door open to the second floor. I called Mac's name again and heard a muffled answer.

There he was--, hiding amongst items we had stored there. He told me had had heard police sirens and they were trying to find him. Dusty and trembling, this time Mac had hidden himself.

Chapter 7

THE FAMILY REACTS

Relatives can become an important facet to your support system. Mac has four brothers married with families, but scattered over the country. It is interesting when this debilitating disease appears, and research finds that some patients probably have abnormal genes that contribute to this disease, families can have different reactions.

One brother has little contact, makes few inquiries and seemingly takes a "head in the sand" approach. Luckily for him he lives far away which makes this attitude easy to do.

Another brother makes inquiries through his wife for the most part, and seems to look at the facts unemotionally, perhaps since he works in science.

A third brother inquires occasionally, but the phone calls are always from some exotic location with extensive descriptions as to how much fun he and his wife are having ("you really should travel here sometime") and making it clear he really doesn't want the particulars of our situation but wants us to keep abreast of his activities.

The fourth brother lives nearby and his wife calls often to inquire how we are doing. This brother has also helped me take care of Mac in social situations and there is a firm offer to help if I need him. Their daughter, my niece, makes the same offer.

I'm sure all Mac's brothers are looking at the statistics of what the chances are of contracting the disease if your sibling has Alzheimer's.

Perhaps they don't understand the immense stress of twenty-four hours on duty with an Alzheimer's patient when a few hours of sitting would mean so much.

Everyday I am in touch by electronic mail with one or more of my many cousins who know of our family situation. Those letters mean so much when I have limited contact with other adults and cannot travel. Some of the cousins and their spouses have made special efforts to include a visit when they are traveling in the area.

One special aunt makes it a point to telephone on a regular basis and it is comforting to know she is thinking of us.

The Community Reacts

Because we have lived in this town many years, and this is where Mac established his practice as an engineer, he has appeared representing clients at zoning meetings, town meetings, and on television. Mac also has held board positions for the city zoning commission, as one of the directors of our hometown bank, and as a consultant to the university in urban studies. He has done well with his career.

It became apparent that something was very wrong, and although I encouraged him to hold on to the positions he was filling until his various terms were up, it was impossible for him to continue and unfair for the various boards and committees. He was unable to contribute any more.

When he resigned from the various appointments, I felt the need to shield him from questions about what I thought was an embarrassment of a brain-wasting disease that was going to change our lives in such a momentous way. People, however, have been kind.

If I have Mac with me, most people always speak to him and ask him how he is. If I am alone, they are concerned and ask about my health and well-being. Most of the social problems are mine to overcome. I fear that Mac won't use the correct eating method in a restaurant, or people may stare if he rides in the back seat while I am driving.

One day, Mac wandered away from the house and when I realized he was missing, I went out to look for him. I saw him across the street, three doors down coming round the corner of the owner's garage. Not only do I feel embarrassment, I acknowledge the fact that the neighbors would not appreciate someone wandering around their property. I cannot be sure Mac would not use their shrubbery for a public restroom.

The leader of our Alzheimer's Association had another approach when I told her of my concerns. She said, "Well, they will just have to deal with it." I must rearrange my thinking. Who owns the problem?

I appreciate the effort acquaintances have made to continue talking with Mac if they see us in a store. I appreciate the fact that the local barber, when I told him of Mac's problem, assured me he always tries to take care of his old customers, and if I gave Mac a bill, he would see that Mac got proper change. Our town has so far been a very caring one.

One very large corporation has been unrelenting in harassment. Years ago, Mac had signed with this company for a cell phone. For ten or twelve years, this company received their payment for services rendered each month on time. When I called the company to cancel the phone, they told me they would be unable to do this, as they would have to speak directly to Mac who had signed the original papers.

At this point, I explained his disease and told them he would be unable to come to the phone but, my son had power of attorney, and I would ask Bret to write them a letter.

This company representative informed me they do not accept "power of attorney". I would have liked to question this, but instead I asked them what they would like me to do. Their request was a letter from Mac's physician, certifying that Mac suffers from Alzheimer's disease. (So much for their keeping our medical records private.)

Our daughter came to our rescue and upon receiving the appropriate telephone numbers, made some calls of her own. She, though she lives across the country, typed the required letter for our family doctor, and faxed it for signature. Our doctor cooperated and we sent the letter to the phone company that would not accept power of attorney but wanted access to medical records of our patient.

The next week, nevertheless, the harassing phones

calls started to arrive again. Again, the representative stated how he would have to receive the cancellation from Mac himself—on and on they repeated themselves.

Again, I called my little mover and shaker in the South, and my daughter made it very clear, about what our family required. It looks as if our account is cancelled!

Chapter 8

"DEAR CAREGIVERS"

Today I received a letter that began "Dear Caregivers."

Here is a label I never thought I would wear. All the years of our marriage, Mac had experienced very good health. I can remember feeling angry when he had a migraine or the flu. My expectations were for him to be strong and take care of me. Throughout our marriage, he has had many opportunities to do just that and has done so without any complaints.

Neither of us knew much about Alzheimer's or dementia of any kind. My only experience with dementia had been when my Dad lost his short-term memory when he was in his eighties. That, while an inconvenience, was more a source of humor than tragedy. I would ask Dad what he had eaten for lunch, and he would answer, "Now you know I can't remember what I ate an hour ago." Alzheimer's is so different. These patients don't know what time of day it is, or what day it is, or what season or year it is. They don't know if they have eaten in the past twenty-four hours. They probably won't answer you.

Mac has never said the words "Alzheimer's disease." He has never talked about it, nor asked about it even on the way home from hearing the diagnosis. I have tried to protect him from what I knew, and have subsequently learned, about the disease.

On the other hand, I immediately began research into everything I could find via the library and internet and questioning anyone familiar with the disease. No research can prepare you for the twenty-four hours caregiver position.

The progression of the disease seems to be individual for every Alzheimer's patient. Sometimes the slope downward is slow, and at other times, it is fast. Some patients have bathroom issues very early, and others never have the bathroom issues. Some patients have motor problems early, and some never acquire motor problems. It seems to depend where the plaque forms in the brain.

Mac cannot tie any of his shoes anymore, except for his black Air Force shoes, which he ties perfectly every time. Mac retired as a colonel in the Air Force Reserves and was extremely proud of his record. The only explanation the doctor gives is when we learn a task, the more times we repeat the task, the more intense the pride in the task, the deeper the groove in the brain tissue. Consequently, the slower that groove would be to fill in with plaque.

In the beginning, Mac seemed to want me in sight all the time. He would stand outside the bathroom door when I was showering, or he would stand in the kitchen aisle if I were trying to prepare a meal. If he stayed with our son's family while I ran an errand, or if I had lunch with a friend, after half an hour he would begin to wonder aloud when I was coming back and pace the floor looking out the window. He may have been experiencing fear or panic but he never voiced those concerns. One close friend said he could see the panic in Mac's eyes whenever I went out of sight.

Many people who have family members with this disease say they can see the change that occurs in the patients by looking at their eyes.

It was during these first stages that Mac experienced sleeping problems. I would hear him up and about and getting dressed perhaps around midnight and then again about three o'clock in the morning. Each time I would get up and undress him from whatever clothes he had decided to put on, and then, put him back into bed. Before I finally consulted the doctor, I was exhausted. The doctor suggested a sleep aid that was to be used only once or twice per week.

Our family learned that leaving lights on in the room might help. In our case, it did and Mac for a while went to bed with the bedside lamp lit.

Once again, there are theories that suggest eyesight doesn't record forms correctly in lower light, and patients awaken not recognizing where they are.

There is a phenomenon called "sun downing". The patient becomes agitated and difficult around four o'clock in the afternoon or just before sundown. Some researchers feel that once again it has to do with the light where forms take a different shape, perhaps when the natural light changes. Some families close the blinds when four o'clock arrives. These patients seem most agitated this time of day. Mac may become quite angry with someone or something he sees and wander around the house kicking the furniture or swearing (something he never did.)

Often feeding him a snack changes his mood. The local health food store suggested I use aromatherapy by spraying sweet orange oil on the back of his shirt or use it in a diffuser. Sometimes it seems to help.

Especially in the early stages, the victims of this disease will tell you repeatedly they want to go home. They are, at the time, sitting in their own living room or den. Mac would suddenly rise up from his chair and head out the door.

Instructions from our daycare center were to follow him outside, and then gently lead him inside through another door. It is amazing how well this works. Before, I was yelling, "Where are you going?" "You are home. Come back and sit down." Or "Don't you go out that door!" This would bring belligerence and unintelligible remarks from him and anger in me.

Caregivers can gain so much information from support groups, especially if you have a knowledgeable leader. The associations for the disease of Alzheimer's are also a good place to acquire information, although I have found it to be of the general kind. Since the behaviors of these patients are so individual, the best solutions for personal problems the caregiver is having often are found in the support groups for Alzheimer's disease.

The feeling I deal with most is anger—anger when I have no one to communicate with, to tell a joke to, or even make an observation on the weather. I have anger when I have to deal with the business world or make a financial decision and I have no partner to consult. Anger appears when I have to meet social obligations alone. Taking Mac with me means watching his every move and explaining his disease. It is hard not to be angry when trying to shop and keep Mac with me while having your other hand pushing the cart. Mac will wander away and I have lost him in a store while just trying to check out with the cashier.

Gone With The Wind

One of my friends has always said that had she had the freedom of time and money to do anything she liked, she would have been a collector. She loves putting together collections of many things in this world and has done so since she was a little girl. She collected salt and pepper shakers, thimbles and pewter sculptures. Her husband and mother enjoyed the same passion for collecting but chose items different from hers to collect. Now, she has many of her mother's collections to enjoy.

Instead of collections, per se, I have always wanted to see how long we could make an object useful either by refinishing, refurbishing, or restoring its use in some manner. Another friend has lovingly restored all her in-laws' furniture which makes for some wonderful memories for her husband each time he comes into their home.

I have restored some of my parents' furniture and have a garage full of items that I would have liked to work on. My older children had Schwinn bicycles when they were growing up. The bikes now reside in our storage area just waiting for some loving hand to refurbish them.

In my linen closet are a few snippets of tatting my mother made stitch by stitch—the only needlecraft I ever saw her work with, and one I have never been able to master. I would like to display them by framing them on a piece of velvet.

I have thought old books with no apparent value except sentimental value could be cut out to hold a wonderful miniature scene reflecting the title of the book as the theme perhaps using some of Mac's or my old textbooks. Before his diagnosis of Alzheimer's, Mac and I had worked some in miniatures making dollhouses for each of our granddaughters and a beach house in miniature about which we created an elaborate story.

Mac and I have spoken many times of how we would take each item that held emotional ties for us and, hopefully memories and knowledge of our family tree for the grandchildren later on, and write a little vignette for each piece making it more meaningful for the recipients of the items.

Mac and I have acquired some small collections during our forty some years together. Those earthly delights need to be catalogued with notes as to where, why, and how we came to collect them.

Painting and woodworking with my scroll saw were newer hobbies I was trying to learn. Sewing and needlecrafts have always been de-stressors for me. When I was a young person, I played the piano. Mac played the drums and trombone. Before he began losing his memory, Mac and I had thought it would be fun to use our son's recording equipment and record some "jam" sessions for a good laugh for posterity.

Time, now, I use for doing the work, or trying to hire people to do the work, that two people used to share in this household. After caring for Mac on the days and

nights he is home, I have no energy for crafts or hobbies.

Thoughts of those activities become merely a sigh
here and there.

Mac does not find anything fun or funny anymore
and rarely smiles. And, our "once upon a time" plans
for restoring, refurbishing, and reclaiming memories
from our family tree have sadly all been put into storage.
Alzheimer's disease has not only made them elusive, but
has made them forever "gone with the wind."

Chapter 9

RAIN, RAIN, GO AWAY-

It was raining hard and my son and I had a hard time finding the office of the lawyer who specializes in elder law. We had gathered our papers and had our questions ready to play the "what if" game.

"What if Mac has to enter a nursing home soon? What if Mac doesn't have to enter a nursing home?"

What if Mac has no major physical problems for years to come and I do? What is the best spending plan for the assets we have, the best plan for Mac, or the best plan for me?

The middle-aged lawyer impressed me with his knowledge of these situations, and the various federal, state and county laws. For an hour and a half, he gave us his best information, and Bret took copious notes. I sat there trying to comprehend it all, contemplating my future, and realizing one has the best choices being very poor or very rich in this country.

With a disease that gives you no clues as to a time-line or knowing which section of brain activity will be affected next, it is hard to plan for your patient's future. Will Mac continue to be ambulatory? Will he still be able to eat the food put before him? Will his disease stabilize and remain at this level for another twenty years? Will I be able to care for him day in and day out without ruining my health?

The county in which we live has different and stricter laws than the next county only four miles away. Every year, our country and state reviews state laws concerning Medicaid and tightens them. The evening news stated that if your spouse is diagnosed with a terminal disease, and you are in retirement, the average couple would spend sixty percent of their assets within the first two or three years after diagnosis.

There is a term called the "spend down" which is used when applying for any aid from the military or government sources. This "spend down" makes sure you have very limited assets when you apply for aid, or you might be denied your application.

Accounts and gift giving are not the answer as these are tracked backwards five to ten years. There are limits of what your gift giving activity can consist. Each year the laws for eligibility for aid change.

Long-term care insurance is a possibility for some. It is only a bargain if you think about this early in your life. Long-term insurance is in its early years and you must choose well and read the fine print carefully. If you wait until your diagnosis is given, it is probably too late to sign up for this type of insurance. Part of the problem is the unknown about this disease. No one can predict the time-line for each patient's decline.

We, as a family, must design a plan of action. It appears most of the care giving will fall upon me. We will spend our assets for occasional outside help. A consultation with a professional who deals in these situations, perhaps while your loved one is still able to help in the decisions, is something that should be high on your list of priorities to be considered soon after diagnosis.

As my son and I left our consultation, the rain had stopped, but I came away feeling I am treading water and just keeping my head above floodwaters.

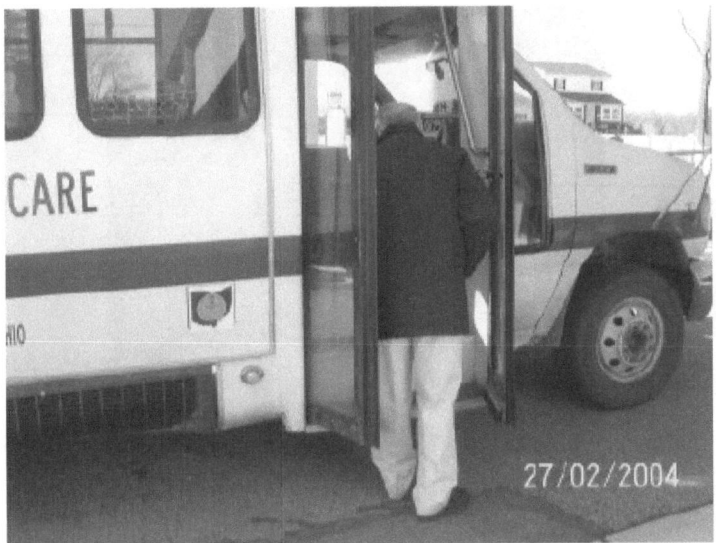

Mac entering daycare bus from daycare center

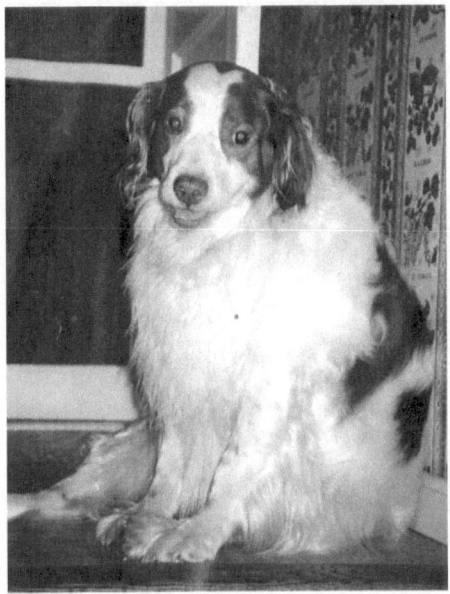

Freckles – faithful friend for fourteen years

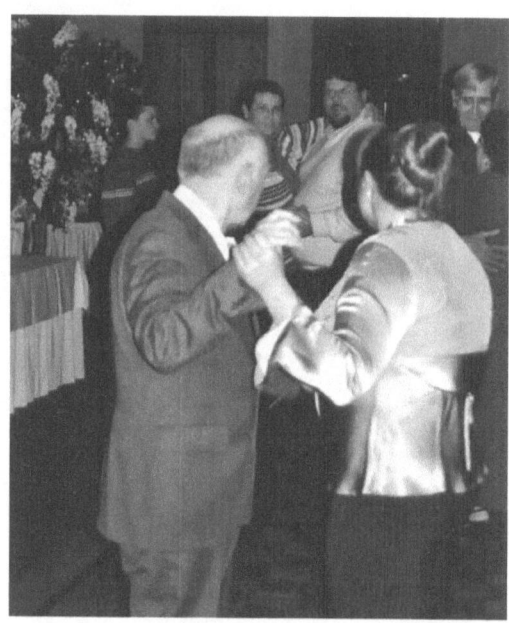

Mac and granddaughter dancing at the family wedding

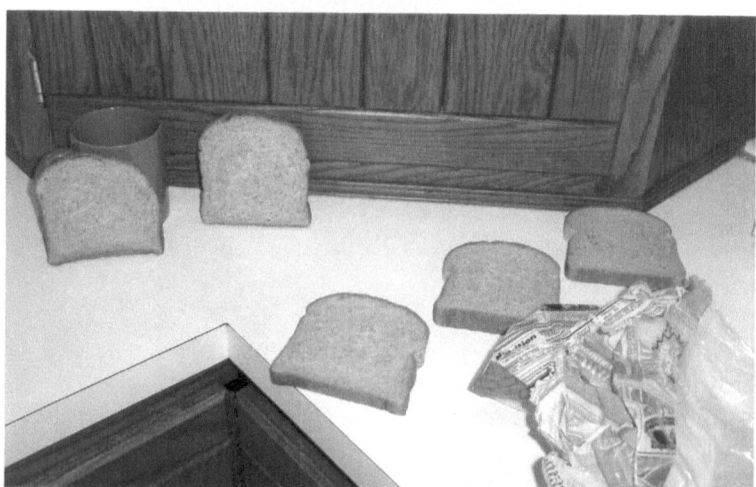

Bread laid outside wrapper on counter in artful pattern

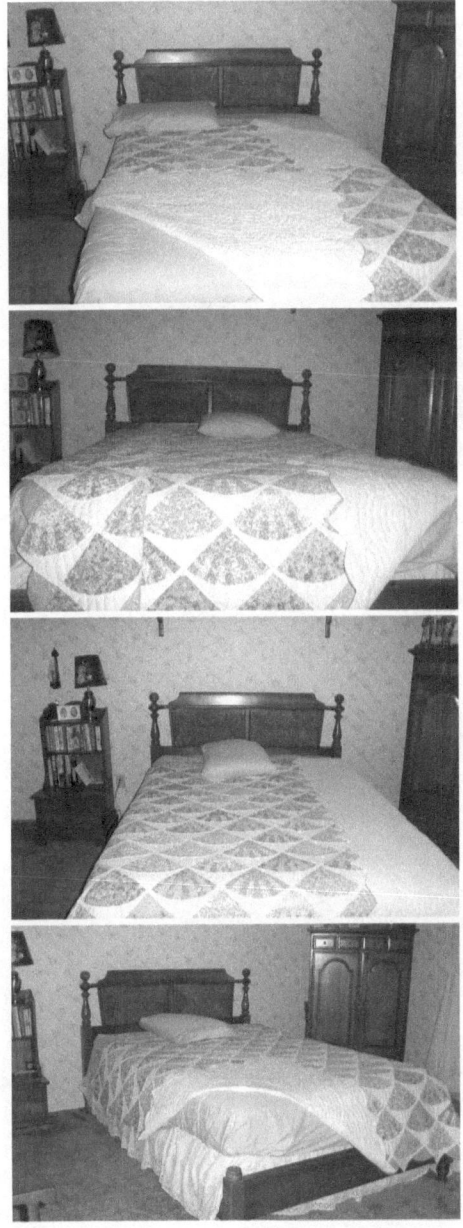

Each day he placed the quilt a different way

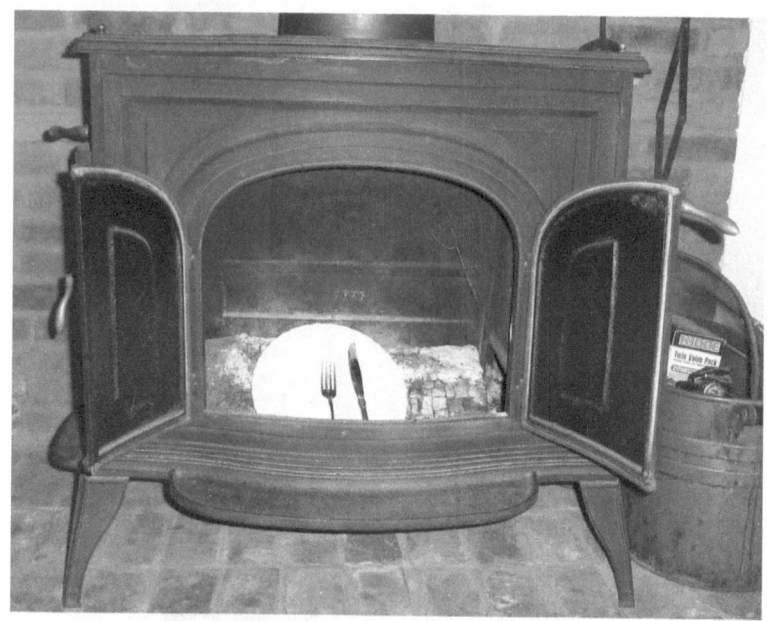

Dishes placed in the fireplace

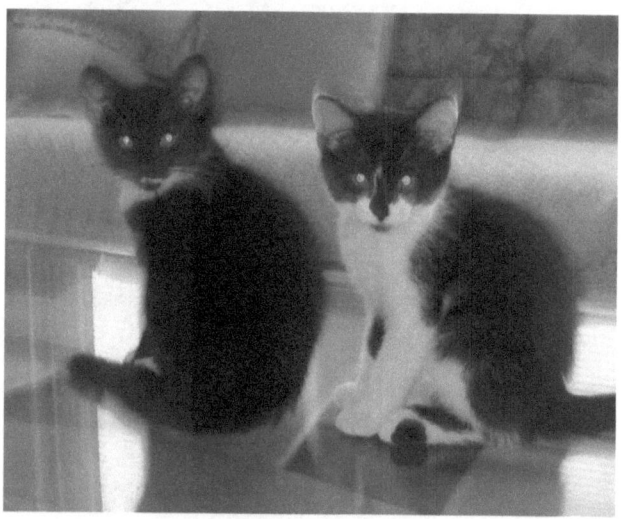

Jake and Sadie

Chapter 10

THE WINDFALL

Fall is fast approaching and the leaves will soon be drifting down but another kind of windfall came our way this week. The Alzheimer's Association had suggested a year ago that I apply for a caregiver's grant. The woman explained that there was a waiting list but if the monies continued to fund the grant, the wait would be worth it.

Last week there was a message on my answering machine from the association saying that they would like to assess Mac's condition, perhaps qualifying him for this grant. Yesterday the case manager visited.

She was a very personable spirit and her questions proved she understood the problems involved in care giving. She asked if I were ever angry about the situation. She queried about my social life (did I have one of any kind?) and how much time the children gave to the situation here at home. She asked if Mac ever held conversation and what tasks he could perform on his own.

At the end of her visit she told me that my grant would help pay for Mac's daycare and transportation until the end of the year. After that, she will again fund some of his daycare and transportation depending upon the state funding of the care-giving grant.

When she left, she handed me a resource guide from our state. It included addresses, phone numbers, web sites, and explicit instructions on how to reach help for your needs either for the patient or for the caregiver.

Former First Lady Roslyn Carter said, "There are only four kinds of people in the world: those who have been caregivers, those who are currently caregivers, those who will be caregivers, and those who need caregivers." Case managers such as ours help us "ease on down the road."

I learned that fifty-two million informal and family caregivers provide care to someone aged twenty and over who is ill or disabled. Five million informal caregivers provide care to someone age fifty or older with dementia. Three-fourths of all caregivers are women. The values of the services these caregivers provide free are estimated to be at least $194 billion each year! This information comes from the National Family Caregivers Association and Family Care America. Alzheimer's disease is the third most costly disease in America following heart disease and cancer.

Should Mac not be able to attend daycare, this particular grant will help me with homecare. However, should he live in an assisted living facility, financial aid would need to come from another source, because now an institution would be providing the "care."

Viewed from afar, these statistics may seem like just so much information. If the scene is from your window, every word is a lifeline for the caregiver.

Chapter 11

DECISIONS, DECISIONS

In my private counseling practice, I tried to give my clients some reference points using water. I would tell them when they saw no way out, one could do nothing like a stale body of water. People could walk by and throw trash and garbage in, and eventually there would be a cesspool or bog. Or, one could become like very fast rapids, acting without thinking about the consequence in the rush to move, becoming dangerous to themselves and endangering others along the way. There was a third choice. You could take a little time to think what the consequences of each action would entail, and what choices would be best for all involved after you gathered as much information as possible about your problem.

As the spouse of an Alzheimer's victim, I must take my own advice. Drowning in pity for me, and for my spouse, whining because of the changes I must make in my daily life is one choice. Rushing to this or that solution with a disease where research gives few hopeful answers can be a repeated disappointment, but it is another choice.

Goals, hopes and dreams have to change when this disease appears, and change does not come easily for humans. I have chosen to gather information from support groups, other families dealing with the many hurdles, and legal advisors, hoping I won't have too many surprises.

The lawyer that lives on my street gave me some free advice the other day. He has an aunt with this disease and his advice was to be sure to remember to live my life without becoming totally absorbed by Mac's.

This is hard to do. My decisions are made by the parameters the disease has set—daycare on Monday, Wednesday, and Friday. You can run errands then, have lunch with your friends, but you must be home by four o'clock when the daycare bus arrives with your loved one.

Laundry, on the other hand, can be done with Mac at home because it takes only a minute to change the loads and you could probably catch him if he wandered away since he would not travel too far.

Paying bills or banking can be done with Mac at home because I can use the drive-through window. Mac enjoys the ride even though he is strapped in the back seat. We must put him in the back seat because he has tried to shift gears while I am driving. He is probably remembering the days when he did the driving.

However, grocery shopping is done more easily when he is in daycare. Catalogue shopping and internet shopping have been so helpful for me.

Our sons need to put the car through the carwash as this procedure frightens Mac, even though in his engineering days, he had designed carwashes.

There is the question of homecare versus nursing home care. When there are no physical health problems and patients are still ambulatory, decisions become more difficult. These decisions are still ahead for me and I must have survival instincts for both of us.

Hummingbird House

Hummingbird House has such an inviting name but the outside of this building is businesslike in appearance and doesn't live up to my mental image of the name. You must ring the doorbell, and step inside the outer entry-way where a staff member will come to let you inside the inner door. Hummingbird House is a secured home for the memory impaired.

I was to meet the director and manager for a tour and interview for possible respite care for Mac, and if needed later, assisted living accommodations for him.

The staff was friendly and the atmosphere was homey. Everywhere was overstuffed furniture and the interior decorators had accomplished their mission. The bedrooms came in three different sizes. There was the private suite, a companion suite, and a companion cozy suite. Each had private baths and for every six or eight rooms, there was a small living room with TV and read-ing material.

There was a small library and three dining rooms, each appearing just as if they were part of someone's home. Each six or eight rooms had an outdoor court-yard, secured of course, and planted with flowers that the patients who lived in Hummingbird House had planted. There was plenty of comfortable lawn furniture.

The manager told me the home is open twenty-four hours and if I became anxious at two in the morning, I would be free to knock on the door or telephone the facility to check on my spouse. Without making a formal assessment, the management felt Mac would be a perfect client for assisted living in this facility for the memory-impaired.

This is not a place for nursing care so the environment is much like a home. Staff does not wear uniforms and patients are free to walk the whole facility. A gentle golden retriever lives there with a couple of bright colored cockatoos in their cage.

When I sat down for the interview, I was thinking that any good salesperson or marketer would try to sell through approaching your senses as well as try to connect a history with the client. That is what happened as the director invited me to stay for lunch at the home. Of course, there was the tour so I could see the place for myself. He pointed out that it was a serene place and usually very quiet. Three out of five of my senses approached.

The director was very good at connecting by sympathizing when he spoke about trials that I am experiencing such as Mac using inappropriate places for a bathroom, or asking about Mac wandering. He was also adept at finding information about our finances such as using the statement, "I'll bet you and Mac have your home paid for", or "since Mac was in the military reserves for such a long time, you probably receive a pension."

What this makes you realize is in the end these people are selling a service. While the care will be there for your loved one, it is not out of the goodness of their hearts. These professional caretakers are paid for this care. This is their job and they do it kindly and efficiently. You must adjust to these facts.

The fact that I might put Mac into a facility is so sad for me. It marks the end of marriage and our life together as he and I have known it. I have to deal with the guilt feeling that I should be able to care for him the way he has cared for our family and me these many years.

But it is becoming more and more tiring for me and I often feel exhausted at the end of the day but still must listen and watch for him all through the night.

I think I have been very accepting of this disease as we confront each problem. Nevertheless, this has become the one-step that has made me really feel the shock and trauma of how devastating this disease can be. However, I do have a plan.

First, I will visit other facilities before making a choice. Second, I plan to use their respite care for six or so months for a weekend per month. I hope this will help Mac make the transition easily if we need to use the care full time. Since this disease has no predictable pattern of decline, the weekend respite may last longer.

Last night when Mac came home from the daycare center, I told him I had looked at a place where he could take a vacation for three days at a time. He seemed to like the idea.

Finances were discussed with the manager and he seems to think Mac's military service may render some funds available if he needs full-time care. But there is a mound of paperwork and applications may need to be submitted many times before approval is given I was told. The director said, "The trick is to be persistent."

That is good advice…I must be persistent against this disease and rise to the challenge.

I have told the children of my plan for their Dad, and they have been very willing to try it. There has been another reaction from Mac's brothers. There was no verbal disapproval except for the tone of voice when they asked, "Would you leave him there all the time?"

Yes, this is what assisted living is—living somewhere else where the patients are constantly assisted in their daily activities. My rational self tells me that it is wonderful that we have such places for these patients and this is exactly what Mac needs. My heart says how cruel Mac can't be at his own home where he has lived for thirty some years and enjoyed success in his career and parenthood.

How cruel that I, his wife, cannot continue to keep him in his familiar environment with all the comforts at the address he and I call home. How hard to take the "next step."

The Question of Medications

In the beginning, Alzheimer's may progress slowly and during this period, there are medicines that may slow the rate of decline. Every memory loss, as soon as the victim or family realizes it is happening, should be investigated. Many of the memory problems have help for them, and if a patient receives a diagnosis of Alzheimer's early enough, the medicines available help the most when in this early stage.

Physicians seem to take different approaches with some being very aggressive and others taking a more conservative approach. Perhaps they take their cues from the family members since there is no cure, and we are stumbling at best in treating this disease.

At one support group meeting of family members, all families there, with the exception of two or three, had discontinued all medications. They felt it was an unnecessary expense since their loved ones had passed the beginning stages of the disease and no improvement had shown when they administered the medications. The only medications these families felt the need to continue were those for agitation or depression. These medicines help with the "sun downing" effect which occurs at three or four o'clock each day.

Some states have laws prohibiting chemical restraints in clinics and nursing homes. Many doctors are reluctant to prescribe "nerve" medicines because of these laws. Two physicians told me that the only time they prescribe such medications are if they need to change the patient's environment such as putting the patient into a nursing home. Then the doctor would prescribe tranquilizers only during the adjustment period.

Evidently, these medications are very hard on the kidneys of older persons and sometimes make it hard for them to retain their balance, so they try not to prescribe them on a regular basis.

Here is another dilemma for the caregiver, the patient, and doctor,—balancing medications and the unacceptable behaviors.

Part III

LIVING WITH ALZHEIMER'S

"I am beginning to learn that it is sweet, simple things of life which are the real ones after all."

Laura Ingalls Wilder

Chapter 12

PROBLEMS, SOME SOLUTIONS

Not Your Colonel's Country Club

In the beginning, I thought I could handle this disease all by myself. My picture was of a cooperative older person who would appreciate my efforts to make him comfortable, serene, and emotionally secure as this disease progressed. I had visions of keeping up on the latest research, supplying perfect nutrition, and stimulating Mac's cognitive skills.

When it became apparent to our children that I needed a break on a regular basis, they suggested I start looking for a daycare facility for Alzheimer's patients. Guilty, was my first thought. I was guilty because I was pawning off the care taking onto someone else. I felt guilty because I was wantonly spending big sums of money for my selfish needs of wanting a break, or at the very least, an easier time of running errands. When I found myself becoming angry and staying angry on a daily basis, I knew I was like a stick of wood being whittled a little each day by this disease and this stick was about to snap.

I narrowed down the daycare centers in our area to three that I planned to visit. I happened to notice that one of my choices was having an open house for their new daycare facility so I marked that on my calendar as the day to visit there. The next choice was in a town nearby. I had a telephone interview scheduled for that one. The third choice was just across the main avenue of our town and connected to a large assisted living compound.

The telephone interview was informative and the woman conducting the interview was pleasant. She answered all my questions and told me in detail about their program. I had reservations about the location, which was a wing of a Veteran's hospital and I felt the program had strong overtones of an institution.

The second visit to the assisted living compound had a lovely quiet setting. I stepped into a well-appointed office area and waited, and waited, and waited for someone to appear...anyone! Finally, a young girl came by and I told her I was here for information on their new daycare program, which they were trying to fill with clients. This was the month of May and the facility had opened their doors to daycare patients on the first day of March. Perhaps this was a hint that not all was well organized when by May, they weren't full.

The girl tried to find someone who could help me and a woman finally arrived and said she would show me the area where patients spent a lot of time. We walked a long corridor to a room with straight-backed chairs where the "tour guide" told me the patients watched videos every day.

She said that if the patients were able, they just "put them in with the assisted living ones" and they played Bingo a lot. She then told me they expect the patients to walk to the cafeteria where they have their trays brought to them. She very brightly remarked that once per month, the patients went by bus to eat out.

At the open house of the third facility, I was greeted at the door of a new building that was bright and airy. The building had an enclosed courtyard where Alzheimer's patients would have to scale a six feet concrete fence to wander off. The setting for this facility was in the country with roses blooming around the doorway. Inside, there were recliners for all patients with an afghan on each and a teddy bear for each to nap with during the afternoon.

The small tables that filled the eating area each had linen appointments and flowers. There was a nurse, and an occupational therapist. Once a month a podiatrist visited and if your loved one needed hair salon care, even perms, it was available once a week. The nurse kept records of patients' vital signs.

There was a craft room and a room for dancing and exercising. Every morning the patients gathered for news time where they were reminded what day, month, and year it was. The patients would have a hot meal at noon, using only soft foods, and two snacks – one in the morning, one in the afternoon. Every holiday had decorations and a "party" was celebrated. Family members could visit at any time and volunteer if they so chose.

The cost for this facility was the same as for the other two. However, it was farther away from our home. I could transport Mac back and forth, or I could use their transportation service adding quite a bit to the cost per day.

The Antonine Sisters administer this daycare. These ladies explained to me that they were there to help me and give me the care that I needed by taking care of my family member while I took care of myself.

I thought to myself, what an interesting perspective. None of these facilities is your Colonel's country club, but this place of all three I visited, came the closest. I chose this daycare for Mac.

In the first weeks, I transported Mac two days per week. Mac liked going to the daycare center and every day came home in an upbeat mood and smiling. These loving people have plenty of help at the daycare center and have the patience of Job. One Sister has worked in a nursing home, the Alzheimer's wing, for twenty years. She is aware of the nuances of the disease. This Sister attends our support group meetings at the daycare center, which are led by the Alzheimer's Association, and she gives us many tips she has collected over the years of working with these patients.

These days of freedom with Mac in the daycare center made the other days of the week easier to deal with when I have to take care of Mac by myself. Before long, I decided to add a third day of attendance for him.

One day the Sisters notified me that Mac became belligerent, threw a coffee cup at one of the Sisters, and pushed another client. The staff felt that the problem could be corrected if one of their buses could transport Mac. Mac seemed to become agitated when the buses began to fill with clients leaving for home, and I had not yet arrived to take him home. I agreed to try the transport, which would solve the problem, and give me nearly another hour and a half on my "free" days.

This solution has worked so well. Mac enjoys getting

"ready for the bus" which picks him up in our driveway and delivers him there in the afternoon. He feels he is really "one of the group".

My guilt has not entirely passed but long-term, it has helped me retain some sense of normalcy in my life.

Alzheimer's 101

Our patient has not tolerated many of the medications well. One made him very nauseous and he fainted. Another made him dizzy, and he fell face forward collapsing without trying to save himself.

I called 911 and when the medics arrived, they determined all vitals were stable. The medics felt it was just the medicine. Another little pill made Mac so comatose that it required two men to get him into bed. We all agreed never to give him that pill again.

The one medication that Mac has been on from the beginning is an old tried and true medicine that doctors prescribe for schizophrenics on a regular basis. Mac is taking a minimal dose and we have found that adding the second dose in the afternoon is too much. I use an over-the-counter sleeping aid when Mac is too agitated to sleep.

Our doctor has made us aware that these sleeping aids can have negative effects if used on a regular basis. Alzheimer's disease is not an easy disease to medicate with a mosaic of symptoms, and a mosaic of individual reactions to those medications.

When Mac reached forty or so, the inevitable occurred with his eyesight and he began holding the pages farther and farther from his face. A trip to the eye doctor yielded a pair of glasses. Since that time, Mac has worn his eyeglasses every day.

Not too long ago he began pushing the glasses down on his nose so he was peering over the top of the lenses. I thought that perhaps they were uncomfortable on his ears or nose. We stopped at the optician's to have them adjusted, but Mac continued to pull them down on his face.

Eventually I just did not put them on him, and he has never asked for the glasses. We were unable to retest his eyes because he is unable to tell anyone whether this or that lens is best.

Mac's glasses were mostly for correcting far-sightedness. If it is true that the Alzheimer patient views everything in only a fourteen-inch square, looking neither to the right or left, or up or down, then, perhaps glasses are superfluous for these patients.

It has been the same with Mac's dental exams. I take him for his regular cleaning and he has had no major problems with his teeth. The last time the hygienist had trouble keeping him in the dental chair to complete the cleaning. Mac simply got up to leave and his behavior told the hygienist that he had enough of this procedure. He cannot follow directions such as "open wider" or "bite down on this", and I am sure the technician wonders if he will bite her if she angers him.

The caregivers, the attending physicians, dentists, and optometrists, all experience challenges in bridging the gap between necessary and unnecessary therapies for these patients who are not comfortable or secure in these procedures. We must constantly ask ourselves, "What is quality of life for these victims of Alzheimer's disease?"

Someone said that Alzheimer's disease places its victims as close to the "walking dead" as you can get. That seems harsh when your loved one is in the first or second stage.

The first stage has much hope because if the diagnosis occurs in this stage, this is where most of our current medicines can help relieve symptoms and prolong the decline.

The Alzheimer's Association uses the descriptive list below as the stages of progression:

First stage:
1. Forgetfulness
2. Impairment in judgment
3. Increasing inability to handle routine tasks.
4. Lack of spontaneity
5. Lessening of initiative
6. Disorientation of time and place
7. Depression and terror

Second Stage:
1. Wandering and preservation
2. Increasing disorientation
3. Increasing forgetfulness
4. Agitation and restlessness, especially at night
5. Develop an inability to attach meaning to their sensory perceptions
6. Muscle twitching may develop
7. Inability to think abstractly

8. Convulsive seizures may develop
9. Repetitive actions

Third Stage:
1. Disorientation
2. Complete dependence
3. Develop an inability to recognize either themselves (in the mirror) or other people about them
4. Various forms of speech impairment to complete muteness
5. Develop a morbid need to put everything in their mouths
6. Develop a necessity to touch everything in sight
7. Become emaciated
8. Complete loss of control of all body functions

Note: Stages often overlap.
As outlined by Ruth Severience, M.S.

One of the first things my oldest son did was order dog tags with the appropriate information for identification and give them to his Dad. We told Mac he was required to wear them now just as he did when he was in the Air Force. He did this willingly. The Alzheimer's Association has an identification bracelet or necklace for the patient and one for the caregiver to wear that connects rescuers with a national hotline. This hotline is a toll-free number that gives the caller information they need to know such as phone numbers and addresses of nearest of kin.

If your caregiver was in an accident or became ill, and was unable to relay information to hospital personnel, this bracelet the caregiver wears alerts medics that you are a primary caregiver, and they will need to call the hotline for instructions. Medics, police officers, and other help professionals are trained to look for these tags. Mac wears this tag in addition to the ones his son had made.

It is important that the whole family develop an emergency plan if the Alzheimer's patient wanders away or becomes lost. Perhaps one member could search the premises of the family home, looking in attics, or crawl spaces or closets.

A town map, divided for driving purposes between family members and friends, might be of use. Often, this can be put into effect quicker than relying upon city services, partially because these family members know what the loved one looks like and what their habits are, and even perhaps where the patient might tend to roam.

Near the last of the second stage and through the third stage, the caregiver cannot do all the care giving alone. Neighbors and acquaintances who can donate an hour or two staying with the patient, and friends and relatives who can give a day or weekend are lifesavers for the caregivers.

A dessert or any addition to a meal now and then is appreciated. Just dropping by, bringing a fast food lunch and staying for a little chat is stimulation for the patient and a stress reliever for the caregiver.

Taking the patient, if he or she is able, for a ride past where they used to live, or past their former workplace, or perhaps to a lake or favorite golf course gives the caregiver some time to recoup and the patient usually enjoys the attention. Keeping an eye on the patient while the caregiver does some very ordinary chores, (such as mowing the back lawn, or sweeping the floor) is such a help because the caregiver can complete the chore un-interrupted. Ask any young mother about the stress of fragmented time. Helpers can try playing a game or look through family albums, or simply take the patient for a walk around the yard.

For the caregiver who is caring for the patient twenty-four hours per day, seven days per week, the environment can become prison-like. If a gallon of milk is needed, it is impossible to grab the car keys and run to the corner dairy. I have had to remove the handles off my electric stove so if I am out of the room, Mac can't turn the burn-ers on. Others have had to turn off the stove and other dangerous appliances by pulling the switch at the fuse box. Everything takes longer to accomplish even if the task is simple in nature.

I prepare Mac's breakfast and seat him at the table. After helping him take his medicine, I rush to the bath-room for my morning shower. I must finish and be dressed by the time Mac is finished eating. If it is a day Mac attends daycare, then there is the trip to the bath-room and the donning of his hat and coat in inclement weather. One thing stressed in manuals for caregivers is the fact you should never rush Alzheimer's patients. It takes so long for the brain to process instructions, and rushing becomes even more confusing to them. Routine is necessary to minimize agitation and confusion.

The career I wanted most in my life was to run a

household. I felt that every room had a different purpose and like an office building, I would try to run each room efficiently with a goal of overall management like a successful CEO.

When planning my new kitchen, for instance, I worked for weeks counting the steps and drawing traffic patterns to find the most efficient placement for appliances.

Solutions and systems applied to the family household were a passion of mine. I liked the financial challenge of managing a household on whatever budget our lifework supported. Sometimes the challenges were formidable with five children and a husband who all had different needs and schedules. But, we made it work.

Alzheimer's disease doesn't lend itself to systems and logical solutions. A simple task like brushing your teeth or combing your hair can be insurmountable to an Alzheimer's patient. Two instructions at one time (turn out the light and come to breakfast) are impossible. As the caregiver, I put the toothpaste on the brush, put the toothbrush in Mac's hand and turn on the faucet to get Mac to brush his teeth. I turn off the water, put the brush into the holder, and then hand Mac his hairbrush. Turning off the light and taking Mac by the arm, I head him downstairs to the breakfast table. Mac will not automatically sit at the place where I have placed his food. He may sit on the other side of the table. I think this may have something to do with his vision.

I have learned that Alzheimer's patients see the world in an approximate fourteen-inch square. They do not think to look either to the right or the left, nor up or down. Sometimes this can be used to your advantage.

If you have a door that you did not want them to enter, you could place the slide lock at the top or bottom, and be sure the patient would not see it.

Learning this little fact changed my thinking that Mac was just being difficult or stubborn when he would not pick up a tissue from the box when it was clearly on the counter in front of him (but not in the fourteen-inch square of his vision).

The fourteen-inch square factor we use again when I am dressing Mac. Originally, after his bath, I had laid out his clothes in the order in which you would normally put them on—underwear first, socks next, and so on down the length of the bed.

I was so upset when Mac would just stand there, waiting for me to pick up the next item. I often felt he was doing this deliberately to challenge me.

Then my daughter-in-law observed that if his vision comprised of only a fourteen-inch square, perhaps it would be better to stack the clothes instead of laying them in a row. Breakthrough! Stacking worked so much better than my old way.

Alzheimer's victims startle easily as their brain does not recognize things instantaneously. If you want them to see something, it must be within the fourteen-inch square.

At times, it is hard to get their attention. For Mac, I make sure I use his name. If this doesn't work, I tap him on the shoulder or take his arm. I have wondered about his hearing. I don't think he has a loss, but Mac doesn't seem to know where the sound is coming from.

If he has his back to me, and I call his name to come, he goes the opposite way. He cannot seem to understand if he is upstairs, and I call him to come down, that he must descend the stairs.

When he was dressing the other morning I said, "Put on your jeans." He replied, "I didn't hear anyone scream." I cannot be sure he heard scream when I said jeans, or was just talking.

Alzheimer's patients often hear voices and see other people that we don't see. Mac often talks to others especially when he first arises. The medicine he takes helps with the hallucinations.

The Garbage Man Cometh

For some reason, taking out the garbage has always been a tense moment in our house. As they were growing up, the boys were either supposed to do it, and didn't, which never made Mac happy, or I would remember that no one had done it. Now it was dark or worse yet, the wee hours of the morning. Taking out the garbage never became a matter of fact in our house like feeding the dog or taking your shower.

It is hard to establish a routine with an Alzheimer's patient and this job, now relegated to me, has presented some special irritations. One day I sacked some leaves and took them to the curb with the regular trash. I looked out my kitchen window and saw there were no sacks at the curb.

Sure enough, Mac had taken them and placed them

all round our property. Some sacks were in the brush pile, some were inside the swimming pool building, and others were stacked along side the garage. And wouldn't you know, the ones thrown on the brush pile had burst. Now there is a tense moment!

Another Wednesday I had taken the garbage to the curb, and again, I found it missing. This time I found the garbage in a brand new garbage holder. It even had wheels. I have no idea where Mac got it. I put it out along the curb with a piece of paper saying, "Is this yours?" But no neighbor ever came to claim it.

Now I must search our garbage before I take it to the curb. If I don't remove the dishes quickly enough when Mac is finished with a snack, they may end in the garbage can.

Unpaid bills have found their way into the garbage sack and, so have socks and clean underwear taken directly from the dresser drawers.

I cannot lift the heavy sacks so I have learned to take the garbage to the garage oftener. And I have made use of that little red Radio Flyer wagon that belonged to the children. I'm so glad that forty years ago Mac and I decided upon the wagon with the large tires and wooden sides. It is just the thing to wheel those garbage sacks to the curb.

A Piece of Paradox

It was a little piece of paradox when the Sisters telephoned to ask if I had administered a sleeping aid to Mac the night before. I assured them I had not and they reported that Mac was unresponsive—"out cold" I believe were the words. They have a nurse on duty and that particular day, they had a doctor-in-training at the center plus a class of student nurses. They had checked Mac's vital signs and reported they were excellent, but he was not responding to them verbally or physically. I told them I would be there immediately.

At this point, the nurse came to the phone and told me that she had help that would assist Mac getting into our car, but she felt that I would be unable to care for him at home by myself. It took only a short while for me to arrive at the daycare center. They had Mac in a wheelchair with a Chux pad for a bib. His head was down, eyes closed, and he was drooling. I asked the nurse to call an ambulance for transport to the emergency room.

Transport by ambulance seems to get attention faster and a room faster than if you drive the patient yourself. We occupied a room in ER immediately but it was nine o'clock at night before Mac was in his own room on the fifth floor of the hospital.

Diagnosis was pneumonia and urinary tract infection. Oxygen and the immediate drips of antibiotics, along with the other support medications for a fast recovery were administered.

This was a paradox for me because as scared as I felt for Mac being ill and not able to convey his needs, there was a mite of relief that tonight, at least, I was going to be able to sleep the whole night through knowing he was being watched by other very competent persons. Perhaps I would have respite for three or four nights, guilty though I felt for having these thoughts.

Five days later, the hospital released Mac to come

home with a prescription of very expensive pills. His checkup revealed lungs were clear and he could probably be re-entering the daycare when his prescriptions were finished.

During his hospital stay, a catheter used for monitoring the urinary tract was inserted. That support system for the caregivers at the hospital rendered havoc with the bathroom issues after he returned home—another paradox in the Alzheimer's scene.

The nurses at the hospital informed me that once an Alzheimer's patient has pneumonia added to his medical chart, he is prone to this infection and it can be life threatening.

Mac, vaccinated every year for the influenza, has also received the pneumonia vaccine. I have been told these vaccines are not one hundred per cent effective and good health hangs softly in the balance for this patient. I live with caregiver's caution.

Chapter 13

CARING FOR THE CAREGIVER

By nature I am a pessimist…my favorite character in Winnie The Pooh books is "Eyore" who claims if anything can go wrong, it will. Therefore, I am always pleasantly surprised when a friend calls to chat or lend a hand.

Someone asked me what I do on my days when I see no end and things look desolate. Since my instinctive reaction would be to mope and feel sorry for myself, I must take positive action to counteract these thoughts.

When I first came to grips with my heart disease, my doctors suggested I walk every day. On those morning walks, I started to keep a diary of what I had seen—the first robin in spring, three rabbits eating clover along the path, or geese in formation in the autumn. I recorded the weather and found after a month or so, I had experienced many pleasant events on a simple stroll.

Depression is a common occurrence after a heart attack. I suffered my share. One day I happened to view Oprah Winfrey's television show and she was explaining the positives of keeping a "blessings diary." Every day I would list at least three blessings that had occurred in my life that day.

I might list the fact that I heard from three of my five

children that day, or my electric bill was not as high as I had expected, or I was grateful that I had the means to buy the groceries we needed and could indulge in making a dish whose ingredients were outlandishly expensive.

In only a few weeks of writing in the diary, and re-reading it, you come to realize your life is not just a downward slope. After a few months passed, I saw by turning my writing upside down, the characters had changed from stilted and backhanded to flowing and with bigger loops indicating a happier more centered person doing the writing. There was even a "happy face" in the margin.

Knowing these little exercises will work for me, helps me get through times when I tend to see only a bleak land-scape. Others might find uplifting in the spiritual realm, or in physical exercise. Many times our first reaction is to depend on others to help our spirits soar. It would be wonderful to give the responsibility to others but that often brings more disappointment when "others" turn a deaf ear. Alzheimer's can be lonely for the caregiver, but the caregivers must also care for themselves.

Friends are made by sharing a history of activities, thoughts, ideas and time. The more these things are shared, the richer the history and the deeper the friend-ship. This reflects the efforts one must make to nourish a friendship.

The rewards are great and Alzheimer's in the family proves this over and over again when friends come to the rescue. I am so glad to have my friends take an interest in my well-being as a caregiver and inquire often about Mac's health. Being a friend to someone who has so many needs can be tiring for the friend too, but I appreciate their "Winnie The Pooh" understanding and kindness in this dark and scary woods.

Send Yourself Roses

Alzheimer's patients seem not to see shapes as we do or perhaps they have no memory of how a commode looks. If your patient is male, it is wise to remove potted plants, especially ones sitting on the floor. I have learned to turn my hampers around with the hinges facing the outside. When they face this way, the lids are not so easy to lift.

I keep all wastebaskets hidden or up on a stand. My scrub buckets are upside down when not in use. The louvered doors that are painted white on the clothes closet remain open at night. And, we still have inappropriate events.

Beyond the nighttime watch, I have begun the time-keeping that recalls the potty training of my children or the puppy training of newly acquired pets. Mac has begun to have bathroom issues and it is time to put adult diapers to use. I simply told him this was a new kind of "underwear" he is required to wear. Surprisingly, there has been no resistance on his part.

One can compare this timekeeping to that of the time-keeper for sports—you can watch the game, but must be alert to pressing the buzzer. This is the doctor-recommended plan of taking the Alzheimer's patient to the bathroom every two hours. This works most days for us as I mentally add the two-hour alarm to my daily care giving chores.

The nighttime watch is a little more complicated. Mac arises for the bathroom visit by himself but the other day ended by placing the bathroom rug inside the commode. He rarely goes back to bed and instead, will start rearranging the dining room furniture, or turn on all the lights in the house. Sometimes he will arise and mistake a closet for the bathroom. I usually hear him and lead him back to bed.

I have learned to put a sweeper in front of the closet door that is mistaken for a bathroom and turn out all the lights in the other parts of the house at bedtime. At first, I added nightlights so he could find his way. Then discovering that he follows the light at night, and Mac seems reluctant to go into a hallway if it is dark, or open a closed door when the lights are out, I very carefully choose where to have lights.

A company has door posters available you can use to your advantage such as a poster for covering the door that looks as if it were a library. Other caregivers have found that yellow tape used for surrounding a crime scene or dangerous work sites is useful for preventing entry into inappropriate areas.

At some level in the Alzheimer patient's brain, these barriers signal, "Stop!" Pressure sensitive mats at the person's bedside can signal the caregiver the patient has climbed out of bed. Some caregivers have found that a two-foot square of dark colored cloth on the front of a door camouflage the opening.

When your patient begins to wear the disposable underwear, this can be an added monthly cost. These diapers can be found from one dollar each to as low as half that. Most assisted living homes and nursing homes expect the patient to provide these. On the internet, I found a company that will ship by the case, diapers to my home for an affordable price with free shipping included.

Perhaps your local Alzheimer's Association has contacts for these items and other helps and aids for easing your care giving tasks and budget. My favorite tip in dealing with this issue is to make use of baking soda in the laundry and in any of your cleaning chores. It is a great inexpensive deodorizer.

Not all Alzheimer's patients have these bathroom issues. Some never experience this problem. It obviously depends upon how the disease progresses for your loved one. The caregiver must artfully create his or her own plan to cope with the ever-changing ravages of this disease.

Be sure to send yourself roses!

It's The Little Things

It's the little things that will make your visit to the Alzheimer's patient a very positive one. You must remember you will be trying hard to connect with and stay connected with the Alzheimer's patient. Sometimes that is not so easy with these patients.

Acknowledge that the person is there and be sure to talk directly to him or her. Remember the fourteen-inch square of vision. If you have a picture to show, or a remembrance to share, put it within the fourteen-inch square of vision.

It is better to approach the person front first instead of from the back or side. Alzheimer patients startle easily and are wary because their world is always frightening and new.

Use simple words and thoughts perhaps repeating them more than once or twice but using adult terms. Remember to be patient. It sometimes takes a long time for thoughts to register.

Sometimes it helps to slow your speech and move slowly. Mac is moving slower and slower in doing all things and I feel part of this is how long it takes each task to register even though he may have repeated it for many years.

One example is putting on his socks. He takes a long time to think about which way to put on one sock. Handing him two socks at one time is overwhelming. Usually he will fold them and lay them aside. So I hand him one sock, with instructions to put it on the foot I touch. Then, I hand him the other sock with instructions to put it on the other foot I touch. Dressing Mac in the mornings can take most of an hour.

Since distractions such as loud noises, or busy children, minimize understanding or the focus of your conversation, it is usually better to limit guests to one or two at a time. In many ways, patients of Alzheimer's disease are becoming like children themselves.

They seem to enjoy seeing visitors for a short period but easily become frustrated with the extra noise or activity.

Touch is important to the dementia patient because physical contact seems to enhance understanding the communication. Perhaps a handshake as part of your greeting, or leaving would be appropriate. An arm through theirs to guide them to a chair is helpful. Mac will fold an afghan repeatedly or run his hand round the rim of a pillow obsessively. Perhaps his sensory deficits are less in the tactile area.

Speech is often garbled or nonexistent. If the patient tries to communicate, it is best to just nod and be agreeable to their efforts. Mac's speech is best when he is recalling work he did as an engineer. I'm not sure when he speaks nonsense whether he realizes it isn't making sense or not. Usually I can tell by the sound of his voice if he is frustrated, or just making a comment on something.

If I need him to come to the dinner table, tactile clues help. I point to the dinner table, and guide him by his arm all the time telling him it is time to eat dinner. After seating him, often I must put the fork into his hand and repeat, "time to eat."

After having a guest for an hour or two, even family, I can see it is tiring to Mac and even though he has enjoyed the stimulation, I can sense the relief he feels at not having to search a damaged memory for the right word or behavior. However, a friendly smile or undivided attention for a little while, or a caring touch, helps keep the Alzheimer's patients connected to our world a little longer.

The Pause That Refreshes

A friend of mine, whose husband has had several strokes and has had to make life-changes, as I have, often threatens to hire a moving van and whisk it past my place as we head for the "Montana plains." Her E-mail reads, "I'm leaving today—can you be ready by one?"

For Christmas last year I sent her a publication with page-size, beautiful images called "Montana". She gave me the ads for the rental trucks.

Of course, this is our fantasy for escape when the daily chores of care giving become overwhelming. Our fantasy consists of complete freedom with the expanses of endless vistas in "big sky country" to relieve the stress of care giving which comes with prison-like parameters.

Friends of the caregiver can give wonderful "time-outs" with thoughtful invitations to lunch in a quiet café where the two of you can chat. Or, perhaps the time of year lends itself to a quiet picnic by the lake or in the park, again, where the two of you can talk.

Knowing what your friend enjoyed before their time-consuming and obligatory duties of becoming a caregiver happened, helps you plan an unforgettable few hours for him or her to unwind.

Showing up with a branch of your newly blooming lilacs tied with a smidgen of lace before you walk through the art museum, or bringing brownies with that added extra—a dollop of whipping cream, shows that you are really thinking of them in the kindest way.

Remember, the caretakers have no one to take care of them.

At recital time in our family, I planned to give a rose to each of our little participants the afternoon before their performance. The first floral shop I visited seemed too busy to wait on me. The second place closed on a Saturday for some reason. It amazed me to become aware of how needy I had become when at the third shop the clerk praised me for thinking of my grandchildren in this manner and also called me "dear" and "honey", and going out of her way to add baby's breath stems and a short ribbon to each rose.

She had no idea how much I needed her kind words and caring ways and what she added to my day. I will long remember her.

Lunch with my friends is a time to catch up on all the news I have missed. For me, it is not a time for dwelling at length on my sorrows and complaints. I need to know that my old world filled with recipes, antiques, and new yarns for knitting are still there. I need to hear about my friend's family and her concerns. I need to have the opportunity to voice my ideas about issues in our town and nation.

Other caregivers, however, may need a listener to vent their frustrations, their worries, or confusions. To help your caregiver friend experience a balance in his life by contributing some delightful escape for an hour or two, just takes some appreciation of how they enjoyed their life before the "diagnosis" and subsequent "duties".

Many times the caregiver is a man trying to care for his Alzheimer's diseased wife. A game of golf, or perhaps an evening at the ballpark, or simply a brew shared at the local pub where some of his friends gather might be a wonderful break for him. A son or daughter caretaker might enjoy a few hours eating the baklava specialties, or Italian cheese puffs and meeting friends, strolling and munching their way through the local festival.

We caretakers haven't many hours we can be away

and simple pleasures that don't require special thought about dressing for the outing, or special finances, are outings of the best kind.

The basic need of the caregiver is feeling a sense of control and purpose in his own life. To let Alzheimer's disease take over the life of the caregiver, allows the disease two victims. Home health care workers have numerous stories about the heroics of families caring for their loved ones.

Friends can be heroes too, in giving comfort to the caregiver, adding humor to some difficult situations, and assuring them that feeling angry and frustrated sometimes is only human. Friends can renew a caregiver's energy-- and provide a little dream of "Montana."

Chapter 14

HELP FROM THE PAST

Hand In Hand, Friends Forever

When I was in the fifth grade, we had two grades per room. Sitting on the sixth grade side was a lovely girl with dark skin and dark hair, almost a Grecian look about her. She became my best friend. We shared all those things that little girls of that age talk about and notice.

When I was in my late teens and twenties, Barb was still my best friend. We went to the high school proms at the same time, and off to college at the same time. We also were in each other's wedding.

When our husbands were both in the Air Force and we were living far apart busy raising our babies, we did not see each other. The occasion arose for us to reconnect after the service years, and it was as if we had been apart for only a week or two. We started right where we left off sharing the things that women in their child-raising years share.

Now in our retirement years, Barb is still my best friend. With E-mail, we are in contact three or four times each day even though we live many hours apart. We share our daily lives just as we did in fifth grade and Barb is a friend of the very best kind—nonjudgmental and so supportive at a time when that means so much to me.

Mac and I have lived in three separate locations in our town, and in the second location, we had neighbors about our age. They became such good friends we even took some vacations together. The men were in the Air Force Reserves together, and our families enjoyed the same things.

Shortly after we moved to another side of town, our neighbors moved also and chose to build a home where our back yards connected. Nevertheless, life goes on, and after a time our neighbors divorced. However, Lee and I have remained friends even though our lives have changed.

We still manage to have lunch and do a little shopping together, share some knitting patterns, and complain about our lack of computer literacy. We reminisce about our former weekend shopping trips to Canada and the fun we had.

What activities we plan now can only take place the days Mac is in daycare. Weekend shopping trips are out of the question.

I have made it a point to renew friendships with some old friends from high school. It has been fun to share old memories with them and hear about their daily lives. One thing a spouse of an Alzheimer's victim loses, is the memory sharing. It is a sad loss. It is important that caregivers keep in touch with their friends, as friends become an important part of your support system.

Alzheimer's can be such a mosaic. Just when you are depressing and stressing over the lost memories for your spouse and pining for someone with whom to share your thoughts, a telephone call comes or a visitor appears and you have the chance to remember and chat about the good times.

Today, my call came from a roommate from college days who now lives in a state far away. Her chosen career was nursing so she understood Mac's disease but more than that, she had experienced a recent loss of her spouse with ALS, better known as Lou Gehrig's disease.

In her case, her husband's body slowly died but left the mind intact. In my case, Mac's body is strong, but we have a mind-wasting disease.

I hope I was able to say comforting things because her loss is so recent, but every loss is so personal it is hard to know. We have made plans to meet in October when she returns for a time to our state.

Help From Unexpected Places

Thinking the other day about the difference between people that influence and mold one's life, I thought of all the people who stand out in my memory either way.

My earliest memory of someone who molded and influenced my life is my grandmother who came to stay with our family when my mother returned to teaching. It is a pleasant memory of warm smells from the kitchen when I came into the house from school, and taking the time in the evenings to play "Authors" with me, a favorite card game of mine at the time.

Of course, parents are the standout influence for most children and teachers fall not far behind. Institutions can be molders too, such as a church that provides guidance in your growing up years. Wouldn't it be interesting to have a tool where we could measure whether your life experiences will be chosen more by the gene pool you inherited, or the persons you meet in your environment and persons from who you choose to learn?

An acquaintance of mine worked in social work. She was remarking to one of her clients that she just could not understand how this client could keep going with all the tragedies and woe that she was experiencing. The woman answered, "Well, Missy, if a woman's house is clean, she can stand mos' anything!" I have thought about the truth of her statement so often. It is an element of truth about control that can easily be applied to all parts of your life. Other important influential people in my life, and ones I would be the first to acknowledge, are housekeepers that have helped me over the years.

Mrs. Bartley (we never called her Mary) came to help when the children were babies and she stayed until they graduated from high school. From her I learned that organization, and thinking ahead are the keys to successful management.

A truck had hit Mary while shopping and her injury left her with one useless arm. Mary had married, and was so successful at her career of housekeeping for others, she always had a waiting list for her services.

With one arm, she could wallpaper, sew, scrub, drive a car, and cook. In our house, we eventually forgot Mrs. Bartley was working under a physical handicap.

Mrs. Bartley pointed out that if she came at the end of the week, the children would be home for the weekend and I would live with the messy house until the next weekend. She wanted to come to work the first of the week, so I would live in a clean, neat home for the rest of the week while the children were in school.

Mary took my home seriously and decided that she could clean the whole house doing a "once-over" in the morning, and in the afternoon, one room would receive a "tear-down" thorough cleaning. This would eliminate spring and fall cleaning, as every room was thoroughly cleaned oftener than just spring and fall, which to Mary's way of thinking, was just not often enough.

After Mrs. Bartley retired, another housekeeper came to help. This woman didn't take my house so personally, but was willing to follow any instructions for the day. She had collected so many unusual shortcuts that made so much sense, I wondered why I had never thought of them. She went home to needlepoint canvas squares for placing under my canisters so there would be no marks on my counters. I still use those needle pointed squares today.

Our housekeeper was willing to move in with the children for short periods enabling Mac and me to enjoy traveling for a week or so at a time. She, when the children were in high school, did teach them what an "Alabama Slammer" was. And silly me, came home and finding some good orange juice in the refrigerator, drank it right down. On my firm suggestion, the children were not taught about any other "grown-up" drinks.

Anna had suffered a tragedy in her life and had chosen at her doctor's urging to take a little day job to re-enter life. At the time, I needed some help with the monumental challenge of laundry for five children, one of which was still in diapers.

Anna came once a week to help with the laundry and ironing. Anna would encourage the children to come to the laundry room and talk with her and she found my youngest son "the funniest little person I've ever met."

He entertained her and today when we see Anna, she asks about him first and ends her sentence with "the laughs he gave me." Anna had the children bring their dirty laundry to the laundry room and had them help her put them back into their proper closets and drawers. This established some wonderful habits with all the children except one—the one Anna found so entertaining. He was the messiest kid on the block and interestingly enough, grew up to be "Mr. Neatnik."

These women have a daily effect on my life as I continually use their no nonsense approach to housekeeping at a time when minutes are at a premium and the challenges of an Alzheimer's patient in the home are monumental.

They could accomplish much in a short time, and knew how to pace their energy to last all day. They showed me how to prioritize my chores, and to budget wisely time and money. I never realized how much I would use their ideas and their outlooks on life to deal with a deadly, tiring and frustrating disease such as Alzheimer's disease.

Chapter 15

UNEXPECTED ANGELS

Angels do not always appear with the golden hair at an appointed time. Sometimes they come with a shock of silvery locks when they are least expected. The voice at the other end of the phone line said, "Little Bit, I promised your Daddy I would take care of you. And looking at your situation now, it seems as if you could use some takin' care of."

When you are on my side of sixty, anyone who calls you "little" anything appears as an angel! Then, in a long forgotten time for a long forgotten reason, this silver-haired angel reappeared to help make good on a promise to my Daddy.

As his schedule permits, this person who has lived alone for the past few years, packs his tools and work clothes in his van and begins the three-hours trip to our town, bringing along comfort and restoration to a tired and stressed household. He will spend a few days mowing our grass, rebuilding our grape arbor, and fixing the sweeper cord in exchange for some home-cooked meals, evenings recalling childhood memories, and sharing a joke or two along the way.

Weary from watching over Mac, and care giving in

general, the arrival of someone who for a short time will "watch over me", restores my spirit and gives me relief in the daily struggles of caring for an Alzheimer's patient alone. For a few days, I can take the time to relax with some deep breaths, to sleep a mite sounder with another person in the house at night, and to enjoy ordinary conversation, a scarce commodity for anyone living with an Alzheimer's patient.

Since our friend's mother was stricken with Alzheimer's, our angel realizes the challenges that one faces and the frustrations one feels every day trying to cope with a disease that constantly shocks you with ludicrous behaviors.

To remain a constant caregiver, I must not become overwhelmed with my task. I must be aware of what can inspire me, to remain focused on what matters, and retain my resilience. Angels appearing in unexpected places in less than traditional ways can provide solutions for doing just that.

Chapter 16

JAKE AND SADIE MOVE IN

This week Jake and Sadie came to live with Freckles, Mac and me. When my granddaughter and I made the trip to the vet's for Freckles special food, the doctor asked me if I would consider another cat or two. It seemed as if a mother and her five newborns were on the doorstep of the veterinary clinic when the staff arrived at work about four weeks ago. Knowing that my cat had died in my arms last winter, and Freckles is 98 years old in people years with diabetes, that has made him blind and deaf, the doctor thought some younger pets might be just the thing.

Brandi and I followed the technician back to the ward to have a view and there they were—two feline siblings rolling and tumbling all over each other. Brandi, a real animal lover, thought we should scoop them up and take them home right then. I asked if we could think it over.

Part of my concern was if I should take on any more responsibility because, in our house, pets seem to have very long lives. I wondered how Mac would react to new pets although he had always enjoyed cats more than dogs whereas I considered myself a "dog person." Didn't someone say, "Dogs have owners, cats have staff" implying that cats were a lot more independent? Of course, that would be a plus. However, I have always enjoyed that doggie unconditional love.

What I have found is that everyone has an opinion about your choices. My daughter-in-law was all for the adoption. One of my cousins E-mailed that she wondered if I were out of my mind taking on more responsibility. One son encouraged me to go ahead and bring them home as I wasn't going to be traveling anyplace and they might be fun to watch.

Another cousin wrote she hoped I had as much fun with these cats as she did with hers. Another son has told me that his family has allergies and he can't be responsible for their sneezes. My cardiologist wants me to have pets always, as pets are evidently a depression and blood pressure reducer.

There are no "on the fence" persons when it comes to voting on adopting kittens.

Bret went with me to move Jake and Sadie into their new home. Mac has slowly noticed that they are here, and Freckles hasn't said a word one way or the other, gentle old bird dog that he is.

Jake and Sadie are called "tuxedo cats" – mostly black, but with definite white markings often in the shape of a tuxedo. Jake is the aggressive one and Sadie is the whining ("where are you Jake? I can't see you or Mommy") one.

Mac is watching them more and more and this morning he actually laughed at their antics... the first laugh I've heard in the past year.

Chapter 17

THE GATHERING

Wedding Weekend

"To have and to hold, in sickness and in health"...my unmarried son has decided to make the big commitment. He and Rosemary have decided to marry in a couple of months. I ordered my dress and I wonder if cadet blue with beading will make me look fashionable. Today I stopped at Hummingbird House to arrange for Mac to spend the wedding weekend there.

Earlier in the week, our family plans to take pictures including Mac so our family photos will be complete. The ceremony will take place in the evening followed by the wedding feast and festivities.

I think it would be too stimulating for Mac and he wouldn't know where he was or who he was with, or what was taking place. The children concur that it will be best to take the pictures earlier, and show them to Mac later. We have chosen not to subject Mac to the rites of the marriage ceremony and celebration that will follow because it would confuse him. I wonder if my son knows the depth of commitment that vow, "in sickness and in health" may hold.

Today I learned the differences between some of the

assisted living facility services. Some are owned and are a part of a nursing facility. The one I have chosen is not in any way connected to a nursing home. If these assisted living programs are part of a nursing facility, the advantage will be if the client's situation worsens, the patient must move to the skilled nursing wing.

In the assisted living in Hummingbird House, I would choose the nursing home if Mac's condition worsened. The motivation in an assisted living place such as this would be to keep the patient as long as possible out of a nursing home.

Hummingbird House will use what in the business is called a 1-assist (meaning one person can assist the patient), with levels up to a 4-assist before considering skilled nursing care unless health problems warrant it.

In an assisted living facility that is directly connected to a nursing home, they may only tolerate a 1-assist or 2-assist before transferring the patient to the skilled nursing wing. Of course, skilled nursing care costs much more than assisted living care.

Some of the questions in the sign-up assessment refer to the extra help the client may need and this adds to the per day cost. Some of our "extras" were the administration of Mac's medicine and assistance with bathroom visits. I had to rate his risk of wandering as low, medium, or high. The basic cost per day covers lodging, meals, laundry, and snacks. The "assists" are extra and seemed to range in cost from one to three dollars. Our total "assists" added to the daily rate was nine dollars.

The interviewer queried me about glasses and dentures. I was thinking that since Mac cannot respond to a dentist or refuses to sit in the dental technician's chair for dental cleaning, and cannot respond to an eye exam, it is of utmost importance to have these exams performed soon after diagnosis while the patient is still able to understand directions.

During the sign-up, I saw a pamphlet by the Alzheimer's Association listing ten signs of caregiver stress.

1. Denial about disease.
2. Anger at the person with Alzheimer's, or that no effective treatments or cures exist yet.
3. Social withdrawal from friends and activities that once brought pleasure.
4. Anxiety about facing another day and what the future holds.
5. Depression, which begins to break your spirit and affects your ability to cope.
6. Exhaustion, which makes it nearly impossible to complete necessary daily tasks.
7. Sleeplessness caused by a never-ending list of concerns.
8. Irritability leading to moodiness and negative responses and actions.
9. Lack of concentration making it difficult to perform familiar tasks.

I admit to experiencing at least six of these but I am realizing there are other people who can provide compassionate care for my loved one as well as I can. When I took my vow of "in sickness and in health", little did I realize the choices I would one day have to make.

The Gathering

One evening after Mac was in bed for the night my telephone rang. A dear friend of mine had been thinking about my decision to put Mac into respite care for the weekend of our son's wedding festivities. With my welfare in mind, my friend felt I would have too many regrets if Mac were not to attend the gathering of family and friends.

If I changed my mind on the respite care, he offered to look after Mac during the ceremony and reception giving me the proverbial piece of wedding cake "to have and eat it too." I would have help if Mac became agitated and the busyness of the celebration became too much for him. My friend would transport Mac home if the need arose.

It was the perfect solution and our friend, true to his word, never left Mac's side.

After the meal, the music began for dancing. Mac was asked to dance more than I was. Our college-bound granddaughter took Grandpa to the dance floor, as did our sister-in-law. As Mac danced, he was smiling. A young woman dressed in blue asked Mac to dance and continued the fun for him. Later she approached my table and told me she worked in a nursing home and can identify these patients immediately. I thanked her for her thoughtfulness in taking him to the dance floor.

One of the catering hall employees came to me and offered to take Mac through the buffet line or sit with him while I filled a plate for him. Here was another person in this world who showed her concern by taking action to provide some real help in a social situation.

Mac's attendance at his son's wedding we recorded in all the photographs of the gathering. My friend, in thinking of me, helped me make the "feel good" decision of having Mac attend the festivities after all. Kind acts of friends and family were in abundance proving once again even though Alzheimer's disease is difficult, there are support systems to help you, the caregiver, and the victim cope.

Long ago, Mac and I were invited to a wedding where the groom was a graduate of the Marcel Marceau School of Mime in France. In place of a soloist before the nuptials, the bride and groom chose to have mimes portray the life of a couple. The mimes playfully acted the springtime of the marital relationship, then artfully caught the nuances of middle life, finishing with the drifting down the path of marriage toddling hand in hand in the winter years. The background music was Irving Berlin's "Always."

Mac and I are toddling true to the tune of "Always." The everyday trials and tribulations of Alzheimer's disease are erased every day for Mac.

For me, I must work to let go of yesterday's irritations to begin each day energized and revitalized. This truly calls for the most creativity of our married years. It is the turn of the season, and I am the memory keeper for two, but the underlying commitment is the same..."to have and to hold, in sickness and in health."

Grandpa "M"

Grandpa M. is a special guy
He loves his grandchildren
As much as he does his wife
Grandpa M is as sweet as apple pie.

Grandpa traveled the world around
This one thing he found
Enjoyment often came to him
Life he knew would someday end.

The disease came slowly to Grandpa M.
He often acts like a child again.
The smile he had is seen no more.
His mind's confusion is shown to all.

We wish you well Grandpa M.
We will always remember you as before
Your cheery ways and comforting touch
These we'll think of from time to time.

Brandi McLean (age 13)

Memory Keeper For Two

ORDER FORM

Please send_____books @ $14.99 U.S.........$_____
Shipping and Handling $3/book.....................$_____

To:_____
Address:_____
City:_____State_____Zip_____
Telephone(   )_____

Method of Payment:
_____Check in the amount of $_____
_____Money Order in the amount of $_____

If books (s) are to be sent to others, please specify names.
"Autograph to _____."

Check and Money Orders payable to:

Madeline J. McLean
510 Bonnie Brae
Niles, Ohio 44446

eMail: MadelineMJUSA@AOL.com

www.ingramcontent.com/pod-product-compliance
Lightning Source LLC
Chambersburg PA
CBHW052244290526
45785CB00016B/1289